The Closing And Opening Of A Millennium:

A JOURNEY FROM OLD TO NEW THINKING

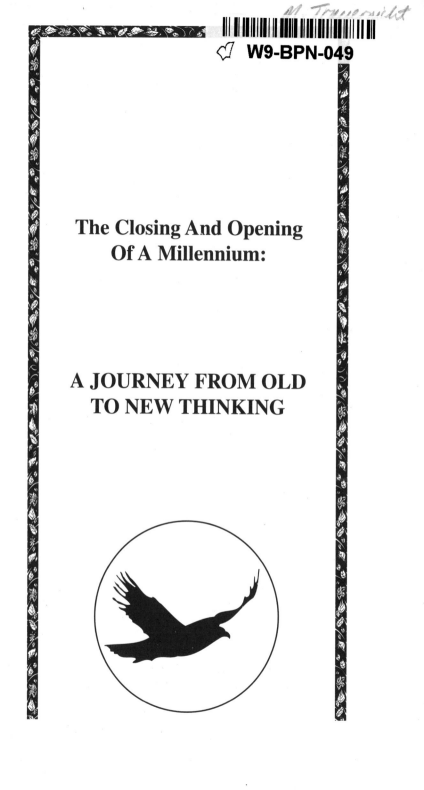

Printed in the United States of America.
Grandville Printing Company,
Grandville, Michigan

Published by:
Practice Field Publishing
100 Michigan Street NE
Grand Rapids, MI 49503
(616) 776-2017

Library of Congress Catalog
Card Number: 95-71362

ISBN: 0-9648264-0-2

---

*Special acknowledgment and appreciation to the
following colleagues whose feedback enhanced
this book.*

Linda Barnes	Suzanne Rogers
Margie Bosscher	Joan Schulz
Peggy Flores	Cathy Schwartz
Carol Glass	Laurie Shiparski
Karen Grigsby	Brenda Srof
Shirley Hamann	Michelle Troseth
Darlene Josephs	Matthew Wesorick
Connie McAllister	Donna Westmoreland
Deb Ritz	Kathy Wyngarden
Carol Robinson	

*A special thank you to Linda Schagel who
coordinated this entire effort including typing and
manuscript layout.*

To God who is life and love,
To my Mother, Helen, and
Father, Morris Henry,
Who gave me life and love,
To my husband, Dave, who shares my
life and love,
To our children, David and his wife,
Fran, Matthew, and Tyler who
expand our life and love.

THE JOURNEY

"People are very apt to find what they seek."

- Emmet Fox

Welcome to a journey into the next millennium. This book is the beginning of a journey that will explore the transition from an old to a new era of health care, a new era of nursing. The outcomes of this journey will impact your health, and the health of your children's children.

No path or map is available. As with most journeys, it is not so difficult knowing where one wants to go, it is getting there that is the challenge. Although it may seem a little strange, there is one criteria for this adventure that is essential for its success: *Please do not bring any baggage.* It will get in your way, increase the risk for wrong turns, and you won't be able to go to the most exciting places along the way.

I am wondering what leads us to take this historical journey together. Is it an accident or the advice of a friend? Is it because someone gave you this book for an assignment? (You might be thinking, "Yes, and it better be worth my time!") I hope it is. Is it because you, as I, are a nurse and you too are experiencing the day to day realities of creating a new tomorrow? Or maybe it is the change, the chaos that surrounds you, that brought you searching. Is it because you are trying to make a decision and you are seeking other perspectives? Maybe you are trying to decide if you want to escape, survive, or lead the chaos that is evident within the health care setting.

Whatever your reason, the road will be different. By the way, if you haven't noticed or experienced the winds of change, then it may be a coincidence that we journey together. It doesn't matter; it is simply a privilege to be with you. Please know, I do not take our time together lightly.

I am not taking you on this journey; I hope we will be going as partners. In fact, the direction and pace we go will depend a lot on you. I promise one thing: You will have a glimpse of the future by the end of this book; and by the end of the series, you will be living in the future you created. One thing is helpful to know right up front: The wisdom in this book is not mine. It is your wisdom and the wisdom of thousands of colleagues who have cared enough about nursing to teach me. I just have the great pleasure of sharing it with you.

I am not trying to speak for others, but trying to share what I have learned from them. If any confusion unfolds as you read, the fault lies either within my understanding or within my ability to articulate my understanding, not in the collective wisdom itself. Please do not confuse the two.

I do not seek to confirm my present thinking, but seek to expand it during this journey. I do not share my learnings for you to accept. I hope to provoke your thinking and to engage your critique and expansion of your personal meaning and thinking about health care and the essence of nursing.

Clinical stories will be shared throughout this series in order to capture the wisdom from the field. The wisdom will help guide us on this journey. The confidentiality of all individuals and practice settings is honored. If you believe you see yourself or someone you know in any of these stories, realize this is not a story about any one individual. We will see ourselves in these stories because they are nursing stories. The universality of each story represents reality across the practice field.

Your thinking, your wisdom is essential for this journey's success. This fact is evident in the layout of the book. The greatest potential of this series rests in the empty columns on each page. These columns are placed for you to jot down your learning, thinking, questions, concerns, feelings, and wisdom.

I will share my assumptions as we travel side by side. You will probably agree excitedly with some, and disagree with others. It is critical during these changing times, and throughout this journey, for you to be clear on what you believe, and with what you are comfortable and uncomfortable. A suggestion is to write down why you agree or are comfortable. When you are uncomfortable ask the following three questions: One, are you uncomfortable because I am challenging or pushing against your basic assumptions? Two, are you unclear about my thinking? Three, is your personal thinking about this issue unclear, fragmented, competitive or reactive? Please put your thinking in the columns. The goal is for you to be clear on your personal patterns of thinking, clearer than ever before. The importance of that goal will unfold throughout this journey.

DECIDING TO GO

"Nursing is a progressive art in which to stand still is to have gone back."
                    - Florence Nightingale

It is good to be aware of the winds of change that will impact this journey. Are you wondering about the change surrounding you? Have you heard, more than ever before, colleagues saying such things as: "I can't keep up with the change around here." "How can we slow down the change?" "Don't go on vacation, who knows what will happen while you're gone."

Change is occurring so fast that many feel the word change is not sufficient, and have replaced it with chaos. What has led to the use of the word chaos? Is it the speed of change or the reaction to change? Changing the word is not troubling. What is troublesome is a commonly seen reaction to all the change or chaos. The reaction is blame. The practitioners are blaming the managers; the managers are blaming the administrators; the administrators are blaming the government. Everyone is blaming someone. *Blame is simply an escape from reality.*

Blame is an attempt to escape from the accountability to live within the change or to lead the change. Blame can be an egocentric response, one in which effects are seen on oneself, not on the whole. Change is not happening because of one person or one event. It is a world issue.

It would be helpful to know something about world issues before starting this journey. At a scientific level, what do we know about the world? The world will attempt to maintain balance just as the human body will work to maintain homeostasis. If there is any imbalance, there will be change or a shift toward balance. What does that mean to us in a practical sense?

Do you remember when you didn't care if someone was cutting down trees in the rain forests? Do you remember when you did not know much about Saudi Arabia, and it really didn't seem to matter until someone you cared a great deal about was going to war there? Was there a time when you did not know much about Bosnia or Somalia? What about Rwanda? Are you familiar with the warring tribes in this region of Africa? Do you think that the genocide in Rwanda matters to our humanity?

Some of you might be thinking, "We can hardly keep our neighborhoods safe; do we have to take care of Rwanda as well?" That is not the question. Do you think that the genocide of these African people matters? Does the killing of people in one place impact our humanity? What are the life lessons to be learned from this genocide, this imbalance?

Let's move closer to home. If you

had a medical problem, would you want to be in Rwanda or the United States? The United States has the best medical care in the world. Note, I said medical, not health care. As you read this, do you think that there is someone abusing the medical system? Do you think there are some health care providers and health care organizations lining their own pockets? Ironically, at this exact moment there is a child dying because of no access to basic immunization. Imbalance? During every minute of the day, tons of food are being thrown away. And at every minute of the same day, people are dying because they have no food. Imbalance?

Change is not being done to us. Emmet Fox (1958) states, "Change is the law of the universe." It is not one person, or a group of people or someone's fault. The change we are experiencing is not merely a nursing or health care issue. It is about world imbalance. When there is imbalance, there is an attempt to offset it.

As this is being written, a friend is in Rwanda. She is establishing a nursing school. People in the United States are sending supplies and helping to make that happen. The effort calls for reallocation of resources, not just fiscal, but all resources necessary for balance. It is a small example of our connectiveness and the shift that occurs because of being connected.

There will continue to be change at an accelerated pace until there is less imbalance. Chaos is the confusing, disorganized period that precedes a higher order. Chaos is about changing old patterns of thinking so as to produce a higher order. Chaos may be a better word to describe what will happen before there is transformational change in health care, in nursing.

Chaos is an invitation to transcend beyond the limits of the present reality. Change is not an option, the process and outcomes are. It is a time of renewal. It is a symptom of hope, the hope for a higher order of health care and nursing practice.

Imbalance is not the only reason for so much change. It is the "time" or "era" in which we are living. Have you ever made a New Year's Resolution? Have you read the many predictions that start appearing at the close of the year? There is a lot of attention to the future during the closing and opening of a new year, decade, and century. It is understandable that there is much attention during a millennium change.

We are a rare generation, one which will close and open a new millennium. Do you remember when you were little and people would mysteriously talk about the magical year 2000? It is a heartbeat away. *The future begins in the minds of those who will create it.* The thinking, the excitement, the planning, the anticipation of the closing and opening of a millennium naturally will bring changes beyond most expectations.

What will be our nursing legacy, that we escaped, survived or led the chaos at the turn of this millennium? It is true that neither of us chose to be born during this time. But here we are! When we were born, we were given a name. At one point in our life each of us made a conscious decision to add to our birth name the initials that describe nurse.

Fox (1958) notes that in the oldest and most read book, the Bible, the name of anything means the character or nature of that thing. He states that the name is not merely an arbitrary label, but actually a hieroglyph of the soul. It is that name, "nurse," that brought us together on this journey. *The question is, do you intend to lead or survive this chaos?* Will it matter if nurses take a leadership role in the designing of a health care system? This generation of humans is calling for a health care system. The changes being made now will not only impact our health, but also the health of our children's children.

There is no quick fix, no one simple approach to bring the chaotic health care system to a higher order. Someone needs to lead and break the present patterns of a "quick fix mentality." That is what this journey is all about. Do you want to go?

WHY JOURNEY NOW?

"This is a world of wonder and not knowing, where scientists are awe-struck by what they see as were the early explorers who marveled at new continents. In this realm, there is a new kind of freedom, where it is more rewarding to explore than to reach conclusions, more satisfying to wonder than to know, and more exciting to search than to stay put."
                                    - Margaret Wheatley

*T*he "C" and "R" Age seems to describe well the present reality of the health care system. See Figure 1. The big "C" word most often heard during the closing of this millennium is *cost*. The big "R" word most often heard is *reform*, or other similar words such as, *redesign, regeneration, re-engineering, or reconfiguration.*

The distressing thing is that many

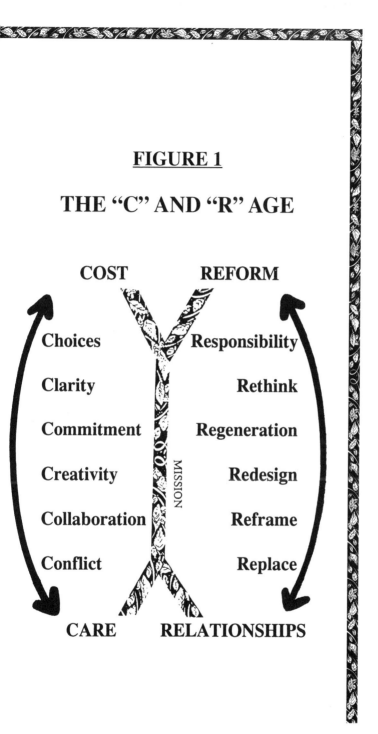

FIGURE 1

THE "C" AND "R" AGE

COST   REFORM

Choices   Responsibility

Clarity   Rethink

Commitment   Regeneration

Creativity   Redesign

Collaboration   Reframe

Conflict   Replace

CARE   RELATIONSHIPS

MISSION

decisions are being made at the *cost* and *reform* level of thinking. Because *cost* is the most obvious "C" and *reform* the most obvious "R", many think that the approaches to deal with the change should be focused at this level. Things that are obvious are often symptoms and when action is taken at that point, it is a quick fix. Change directed at this level of thinking enhances the chaos; it does not help one reach a higher order.

The top "C" *cost* and "R" *reform* are obvious and associated with a "quick fix mentality." The latter phrase is often used to describe the cultures of many health care settings, especially the hospitals. One can get a feel for this mentality by being in a practice setting just before JCAHO, the credentialing body, comes. In what way would you describe the culture? Have you ever heard statements such as, "Get it fixed before JCAHO comes!"

Here is another example of "quick fix" thinking. A new ideal is brought forth at a meeting, and even before it has been explored by the group, the leader reminds the group that these are uncertain fiscal times, and we cannot do this because it will cost too much. The discussion is ended. Or have you heard a leader say, "We need to do this because it will cost less than what we are presently doing." Because cost is the most obvious factor, suggestions to decrease cost get the most attention and are *challenged less.*

A framework for dealing with change that is driven only by cost, is often symptomatic in nature, and not aimed at the root of the issue. Changing from a "quick fix" to a systems thinking culture requires a different type of leader, one who goes beyond the obvious top "C" and "R" and is attentive to the other "C's" and the other "R's."

During a period when old models of thinking are being broken, there are many "C's" and "R's" and each plays a significant role in the formation of a higher order health care system. We are all going to be making _choices_ and will be held _responsible_ for them. The thinking behind our choices is very important. Today the majority of all nurses practice in the hospital setting. It is predicted that this number will be cut in half. Does this mean there will be less need for nurses? No, it just means nurses will be providing their services in different places.

We will be making serious choices about the places we will practice. We will make _choices_ and we will be held _responsible_ for our _choices_. During this chaos we need to have _clarity_ about the essence of nursing as we _rethink_ the whole delivery system. The ability to change the system will parallel with not only our clarity, but also, the individual _commitment_ of our colleagues to carry out the work of _regeneration_.

It is essential to be _creative_ during _redesign_. However, it is hard to be creative when one is exhausted from the practice pace, experiencing fear or worry, or concerned with job security. This is reality for many. The necessary changes cannot be done unless there is collaboration among nurses, the largest number of health care providers in the world, as well as interdisciplinary _collaboration_ as we together reframe our services within new paradigms. Our history is one of competition, not _collaboration._

During chaos, _conflict_ can be expected because typical norms, rituals, patterns, and routines will be replaced. _Chaos is a culture where old patterns of thinking are being broken._ Without the old patterns being broken, there can be no significant change or elevation to a higher order.

There are many "C's" and "R's," but the least obvious and yet, most critical, is at the bottom. See Figure 1, page 15. The bottom "C" and the bottom "R," **care** and **relationships** are fundamental and will provide a pivotal focus from which to develop a framework or context to lead the change and chaos in the health care system. Both provide the leverage for successful transformation from old to new patterns of thinking.

The leverage "C," _care_, is about

our mission, the reason we exist. It is about the service, the health care we render. Clarity on the mission is a critical component of a solid foundation for dealing with change. Cost is nothing more than the symptom of a problem which is evolving because the majority of money is being spent on medical care, with limited resources being available for health care. *The real issue is care, the difference between medical care and health care.*

The bottom "R" is not about reform but *relationships*, the relationships we have with the people we are privileged to serve and the relationships we have with each other and the environment. Relationships are the invisible connections between every human and the universe.

When we enter into relationships, we tap into the unseen energy field of every living thing. There is no life without relationships. A human will die at birth without a relationship with another human. The "R" relates to another major paradigm shift facing the health care arena. It is about the type of relationships and the shift from bureaucratic cultures with hierarchical relationships, to empowering cultures with partnering relationships. It is the fuel for the mission, the journey.

The hope of creating a higher order of health care is rooted in the strength of our care and relationships. These are the leverage points that will bring long term positive outcomes. As Einstein noted, "This is the age old problem with which Plato, as one of the first, struggled so hard: To apply reason and prudence to the solution of man's problems instead of yielding to atavist instincts and passion." Decisions based only on cost and reform are evidence of common atavist instincts and passion!

The success of this journey will rest on our clarity, as partners, on the bottom "C", care, our mission, and the strength of our relationship. When faced with a tough decision, the bottom "C" and "R" will give us direction. *If a decision is being made and it does not improve the care we give or improve the*

relationships _we_ _have_ _with_ _each_ _other_
and _the_ _universe,_ _it_ _should_ _not_ _be_
carried _out._

Why leave now on this journey?
The winds of change are with us.

WHAT CAN YOU EXPECT?

"There is nothing more difficult to take in hand, or more uncertain in its success than to take the lead in the introduction of the new order of things."
- Prince Niccolo Machiavelli

We are surrounded by committed, caring, intelligent health care providers. Yet, the health care system is under fire. There is waste, duplication, difficult access, system complexity, abuse, prohibitive cost, and minimal preventive or other services to promote health. However, the old system is not without its successes. People are living longer than any other generation, cures and treatments that were impossible a decade ago are norms today. No one would deny the need to cut costs, stop waste, and improve the system to better serve the population. That is what all the restructuring is about. Changes are being made all over. There is a flurry of activity. Is this a hopeful sign? Not necessarily.

What can we expect on this journey? It depends on which direction we decide to go. Albert Einstein has given us clear direction for these changing times. He states, *"The significant problems we face cannot be solved at the same level of thinking we were at when we created them."* Simply stated, if we are going to make any inroads, we will need to change our patterns of thinking, our paradigms.

If we continue to think in the same way, all of our activities, changes, approaches, projects, and programs will be quick fixes and not take care of the underlying issues. The work, or activities carried out in the usual patterns of thinking, could be compared to a ride on a carousel in the amusement park. People get on their horse, the music is playing and there is great anticipation. When the ride begins there is noise, they can feel the wind against their faces, it is moving along, and the things around start changing. Then all of a sudden, they start to see the same things over and over again and when the ride is done, they are right back where they started. That is happening in health care settings across the country. Einstein warned us of that.

Fox (1941) stated, "Mind is cause and experience is effect; and so, as long as your mind remains unchanged, it will continue to produce just those effects or experiences of which you are anxious to be rid." Much of the change that is taking place is being done at the same level of thinking that took place when the problem was created. That is apparent in the many new projects and programs being started in hospitals across the country. The often stated desired outcome is to help people do their work faster and better. In some cases the working faster and harder is to meet the institutional needs, not to enhance the mission.

Many projects are nothing more than reforming within the same old paradigms. Reform is not the goal. Reform is trying to make what we have better, which is like being on the carousel. Health care reform could be compared to spending a great deal of effort trying to improve the horse, when in fact, someone was creating a car, a whole new paradigm. We do not need to do medicine better, we need to do health care.

Someone wrote that "Insanity is doing the same things but expecting different results." It is as crazy as thinking in the same old ways and expecting different results. Society is calling for us to improve the health care system. That's why we journey. We can't get to a different place without leaving. Moving faster, working harder, and going in the same direction assures us, as the old Chinese proverb says, that we will end up where we are headed.

How do we change our direction or thinking? First lets explore the old patterns of thinking or paradigms that are driving the health care system and driving practice. The reason this is so important is because the way we think determines the way we practice. The way we think determines the future, the hope for a new health care system. The present system is built on old patterns of thinking. It is no secret that the present system and old familiar patterns of thinking are not working. What are the new patterns of thinking or paradigms necessary to create the future?

Twelve years ago a group of nurses were talking about paradigms. One nurse asked if a paradigm was a disease. What a great question. In fact, it can be, one can die from it. However, it can also be a cure. There are different definitions. Barker (1990) defines a paradigm as a set of rules and regulations that establish boundaries, and tell us what to do to be successful within those boundaries. He notes paradigms act like an invisible filter and one sees things only as they fit within the boundaries. Peat (1993) interchanges the word paradigm with "world view," a way of seeing and thinking about reality and society which drives one's action. A paradigm can be thought of as a traditional pattern of thinking, a personal way of knowing that helps us see, explain, and act in the world we live in.

Paradigms are not necessarily good or bad. Their impact on us can be good or bad. They are powerful. Shifting from old to new paradigms is what Einstein holds to be the answer for creating solutions to problems and the source of innovation. Within the health care setting and the practice of nursing, there are many paradigms.

The hope for an exciting journey rests in our ability to shift from old to new ways of thinking. Before we can change our way of thinking, we need to be aware of it. Covey (1990) notes the process starts with recognizing and admitting our present personal patterns. This process is not done to fill one with guilt, but to free one up to explore and live new paradigms.

One of the goals for this journey is to shift from old to new ways of thinking. Which paradigms are driving your thinking, therefore, your practice? See Figure 2 which lists four of the strong old paradigms that are foundational in the present health care system. It also lists the emerging parallel paradigms. These paradigms will be explored throughout the series.

As each of the old and new paradigms are reviewed, clarify your thinking. Ask yourself which one describes the pattern with which you are most comfortable, familiar, and which one is prevalent in the setting in which you practice every day.

What can you expect from this trip? Something different.

FIGURE 2

OLD VERSUS NEW PARADIGMS

OLD PARADIGM	NEW PARADIGM
Newtonian View	Quantum View
↓	↓
Medical Care Model	Health Care Model
↓	↓
Institutional Practice	Professional Practice
↓	↓
Hierarchical Relationships	Partnering Relationships

OLD VERSUS NEW
PATHS OF THINKING

"The answer lies in the potency of habit; and habits of thinking are at once the most subtle and the most difficult to break."

- Emmet Fox

When exploring patterns of thinking, it is hard to separate one old paradigm from another old paradigm or one new paradigm from another new paradigm. They are connected by similar patterns and often one builds on the other. What becomes apparent is the difference between old and new thinking. The Newtonian versus the Quantum view of the universe demonstrates that point. See Figure 3 for the characteristics of the old versus the new world view.

FIGURE 3

OLD VERSUS NEW PARADIGMS

OLD PARADIGM	NEW PARADIGM
Newtonian View	Quantum View
↓	↓
Materialistic	Relationships
↓	↓
Parts	Wholes
↓	↓
Predictability	Surprise/ Generative
↓	↓
Mechanistic	Dynamic Connectiveness
↓	↓
Analyzing	Learning
↓	↓
Stable	Self-Renewing
↓	↓
Fix -- Measurable	Random -- Non-measurable

NEWTONIAN VERSUS
QUANTUM VIEW

Newtonian View

What does the Newtonian view of the universe have to do with nursing practice and the present health care system? In what way has the world of science impacted our present system and nursing practice? The impact of Newtonian thinking (Wheatley, 1993 and Peat, 1993) is evident in the health care systems and structures of today. Are the characteristics listed in Figure 3, page 32, alive and well in your day to day world? In the Newtonian view, health care and the system are viewed as materialistic, broken down into parts that are mechanistic and predictable. Health, in this framework, is materialistic, therefore the focus is only on the body, not on the body, mind, and spirit. The body is broken down into parts and each part is mechanistic, and predictable. If you want to understand the body and parts, analyze them, and analyze them some more. Things are stable, fixed, and measurable. Does this type of thinking seem familiar?

The Newtonian thinking influenced the system design and the approach to health care. The system within this thinking is broken down into parts, such as hospital, home, extended care, offices, and clinics. The hospital is designed by units that take care of broken body parts such as oncology, neurology, medical/surgical, critical care, obstetrics, pediatrics, outpatient, and inpatient. Things are pretty predictable on each unit, some look at certain parts, others certain age groups, some, the time related needs, each independent of the other, each taking care of a different need.

Nurses within the hospital often did not connect with nurses on other units, and certainly not beyond the walls of the site of their practice setting. Even our relationships developed around the care we gave to people with diseased parts within a certain unit, and a specialty. We are surrounded by a culture that centers on materialistic and mechanistic parts, that are stable, predictable, and measurable.

Quantum View

The Quantum view does not discredit the old, just expands beyond it. To understand health and a health care system within the Quantum view, it is essential to look at the whole picture, not just parts. It is not just about what you see. Many of the critical elements that sustain the world and health are not materialistic, but invisible. The Quantum view is about relationships. Relationships are necessary or foundational to the mission. Health, as the universe, is not about the mechanism of a part, but the dynamic connectiveness of the whole. The whole is not predictable, but full of surprise and generative knowledge.

If you want to understand, the best approach is not to analyze, but enter each day with the desire to continuously learn and explore the changing relationships. The connections are not mechanical, but dynamic; not stable, but self-renewing (to maintain balance and harmony); and not fixed and measurable, but random and non-measurable. The new science, as with most paradigms, is opposite from the old. If we care about health, we can no longer think about isolated body parts that are predictable, mechanistic, fixed, and measurable.

Bohm (1983) stated, "The notion that all these fragments are separately existent is evidently an illusion, and this illusion cannot do anything other than lead to endless conflict and confusion." The science of health, a health care system, and the universe are one. The new pattern of thinking, or new paradigms, gives new and different direction, as well as hope.

A LOOK AT THE OLD
MAPS AND ROADS

"The progress of technological developments has not increased the stability and welfare of humanity."
- Albert Einstein

 $\mathcal{T}$ his journey is not only about establishing a health care system, but also about our personal accountability to a choice we made. I made the choice to be a nurse, my husband a counselor, one son a physician, one son a nurse, and the other son is still deciding. Many different choices have been made by our colleagues in the health care system. Whether we are nurses, doctors, physical therapists, occupational therapists, respiratory therapists, managers, or medical assistants, we have one thing in common. We each made a choice to impact the health of humanity in a specific way, a specific role, and entered into what is called the health care system to do that work.

The health care system has evolved. The medical model drove the system's evolution. It enhanced the development of medical care and institutional practice within a bureaucratic culture. What is this medical care paradigm? Where did it come from? Why is it important to understand it? What is its impact on nursing?

MEDICAL CARE PARADIGM

There was a time when the hospital was the place a person was brought to die. That is the old hospital paradigm. It evolved to become a place where people would come to get help, to restore or improve health. A new hospital paradigm emerged in opposition to the old. During this emergence from a death to a life focus, some important things happened. The foundation for the new hospital was the medical model. Physicians were at the center of this development. The physicians became the leaders of a health care science designed to improve the physical health status.

Everyone knew the importance of this work. Excitement and enthusiasm to continuously improve the physical health status of mankind was fueled by educational advancements and the technological explosion. The rest is history.

The physicians created a structure within the medical model, which supported and continuously improved their practice. The outcomes are obvious. Cures and treatments were discovered for diseases that previously led to death. Common diseases were able to be prevented. Today a person can even get some of their body parts replaced when they get diseased or worn out.

The successes resulted in another major shift. The hospital not only became the center for receiving health care, but also health care was often seen as synonymous with diagnosing, treating, and preventing disease. Insurances were developed and offered to people so that when they needed care, they had financial protection for this expensive, necessary, and utilized service.

The medical care paradigm became the health paradigm. See Figure 4, first column. As a result, today, health is equated with the physical status. This resulted in health being narrowed to an objective, materialistic, physiological dimension. Health is often defined by the medical scope of practice as, "absence of disease." Improving health is seen as impacting the physiological level, such as increasing or decreasing the blood pressure, increasing or decreasing the urine, cutting out a part, or adding on a new one. Evaluation of health status is mechanical in nature. If your body parts are working, you must be fine. Normal life events such as birthing, raising children, eating and exercising, caring for aging parents, and menopause are seen as medical events. To get support for these

FIGURE 4

Old Paradigm	New Paradigm
Newtonian View	Quantum View
↓	↓
Medical Care Model	Health Care Model
↓	↓
"Absence of Disease"	"Body, Mind, and Spirit in Balance"
↓	↓
Physiological (objective)	Human Response (subjective)
↓	↓
Mechanical View	Wholistic View
↓	↓
Life Events: Medical	Life Events: Balance
↓	↓
Fix: "Power Over"	Ownership: "Power Releasing"
↓	↓
Passive	Partnership
↓	↓
Episodic (Short Term)	Continuous (Long Term)
↓	↓
Limited Strategies	Endless Possibilities
↓	↓
Institutional Service	Professional Service
↓	↓
Dependent, task-dominated practice wherein the nursing service is directed by physicians' orders and hospital policies and procedures. *"Doing things right."*	Independent, process-dominated practice wherein the nursing service is based on the individual's human response to the present health status or situation. *"Being there at the right time, intervening in the right way with the right resources to support healing."*

life events, one needs to go through the medical care system, which is not designed to address all of these needs.

When it comes to knowing what is best for the body, the physician and other health care providers are considered the experts because of their ever growing knowledge and technological finesse. In fact, health care providers often are the ones who make the decisions about what is best for the person's body. Within this framework, the relationship between the provider and the person seeking health care has become one of "power-over" or superior and subordinate. This also set the pace for "power-over" and subordinate relationships among the providers.

In the medical care paradigm, the provider makes the decisions or has "power-over," and the person needing health care becomes passive. Passive people make things easier. The providers can see more people and get more things done in a more timely manner when the recipient of care is passive.

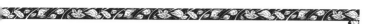

Health began to be seen as an episodic event or a short term issue. The people began to think that if something was wrong with their health, they only needed to go to the doctor or hospital and the "all knowing" providers would take care of it. The competency of the providers, not the actions of the recipients, was viewed as the most important determinant for the health care outcomes.

The outcomes of this evolution and the power of the medical paradigm are evident. The United States has the best medical care in the world. However, the limits of this model have become apparent in the final decade of the twentieth century. The access to the system is not only limited, but when accessed, it is a disease or problem driven framework, not a health driven framework.

The logic of preventing people from getting sick, instead of spending all the money on treating them once they get sick, is beginning to surface. The concept that health is more than the physical status has sent further ripples into the sea of concern. As the millennium closes, health care problems are at the center of political, social, and economic reform. Most of the realizations surfaced because of limited financial resources. Some leaders still think that cost is the primary issue.

INSTITUTIONAL PRACTICE

Before comparing the medical care paradigm to a health care paradigm, it is natural to take a closer look at the influence of the medical model on the services or care being provided, for example, in the hospital.

The limited concept of health as medical care led to a very unique kind of health care service called institutional practice. The hospital, under the medical model paradigm, evolved to become the center of the present health care system. Because the medical model paradigm is the foundation for the hospital structure and systems, the care given is formed and molded within that thinking. This led to institutional practice. I will explore this paradigm from a nursing perspective. The principles of institutional practice are the same for all health care providers. *Institutional nursing practice is defined as a dependent, task-dominated practice wherein the nursing service is directed by the physicians' orders, and hospital policies and procedures.*

Institutional nursing is something every nurse has lived in varying degrees of intensity. Its evolution is understandable, especially in the light of what has been learned about organizational design over the last fifteen years. The hospital is structured to support the development and refinement of medicine. As a result, medicine is improving, with exciting developments and demonstrating excellent outcomes. The culture is focused on assuring the improvement of the physical status of each person. The physicians, the most knowledgeable about the body or medicine, are the leaders.

The other health care providers such as nurses, physical therapists, and pharmacists, were equally aware of the importance of the medical service, and they too focused on supporting good medicine. The system was designed to facilitate the delivery of medical services. The physician wrote the orders and someone else carried them out. The other providers began to be seen as physician extenders whose practice centered on carrying out the physician's orders or meeting the doctor's needs.

Since nurses are the only providers who have 24 hour, hands on accountability for patient care in the hospital setting, their practice was greatly influenced by the medical model. This especially became true as the hospital grew to be the center of health care. More and more nurses were needed within the hospital. As the twenty-first century is entered, the majority of all nurses practice in the hospital setting.

Although nurses provide a unique professional service, equally important but different from the physician, the culture focused solely on nurses fulfilling the medical orders. This reality led to the nurse's credibility being tied to the speed and accuracy of carrying out the doctor's orders.

Because of the organizational design, nurses began to lose sight of their unique practice and vied to be what I call the "Institutional Queen." There could only be one on a unit, two would never get along. This coveted title was not easy to get.

The queen could pass more meds and do more treatments in an hour than anybody thought possible. No matter how many people they were assigned, their beds and baths were always done by nine a.m. They could give a report on a whole unit in less time than anyone else could. The queen was someone people wanted around during a crisis, such as an arrest. They always seemed to have what was needed in their pocket or they had keys to rooms that no one else knew existed and could find whatever was being sought. The institutional queen could not only put

IV's in faster than anyone, but also, in places where most didn't even think there were veins! In addition, the IV's were always on time.

So many nurses got good at these things, a new criteria was suggested. The institutional queen must be able to put a foley and an NG in at the same time....and with one set of gloves! Are you an institutional queen? Are you vying to be one? Do you know one? Have you been influenced by one?

The impact of this medical and institutional pattern can best be understood when compared to the thinking of the new paradigms. The work to shift from the old to new ways of thinking can be sensed in the words of Max DePree (1992), "Success can close a mind faster than prejudice."

EXPLORING THE LANDSCAPE

"There is a call for society to balance the wonders of technology with the spiritual dimensions of human nature."

- Naisbitt

$\mathcal{N}$ew patterns of thinking, or new paradigms, are emerging in the health care settings. The society as a whole is calling for health care reform. The only good news is that the right words are being used, "health care." Refer back to Figure 4, page 41. The difference in the thinking between medical care and health care is obvious. A powerful way to explore the health paradigm is to do it at a personal level.

Have you ever had a day when you didn't feel very well? Was it because your heart, lungs or kidneys were not working right? What was it all about? Do you believe that every human (it's good to start with yourself) is multidimensional? Do you believe each person has a physical, psychological, sociocultural, and spiritual dimension? If that is so, health cannot be "absence of disease." Absence of disease only deals with the physical status of a person.

So, what is health? Health is about the wholeness of a person. Health is the harmony of the physical, psychological, sociocultural and spiritual dimensions. More simply stated, health is body, mind and spirit in balance. Body, mind, and spirit in balance does not mean homeogenicity. Each person's health status is unique. No one person's is the same. Health is not objective but subjective.

The profession of nursing presented a formal definition for nursing in the America Nurses Association (ANA) (1980) Social Policy statement. It said, "Nursing is the diagnosis and treatment of the human responses to actual or potential health problems." During 1994 and 1995 the ANA opened up the social policy for review. Many hours of discussion and dialogue on the definition of nursing took place across the country. It was felt that the 1980 definition adequately reflected the "influence of nursing theory that is a part of nursing's evolution," and no changes were made.

This definition clearly speaks to the accountability of nursing to the health care paradigm. It focuses nursing on the human response. What is the human response? It is a response a human makes out of his/her wholeness. It is a symptom about the health status, not just the medical status, of an individual. It is equally as significant as any physical symptom, but different. It is not a disconnected symptom from one domain or the other. It is a response that flows from the integration of the physical, psychological, sociocultural, and spiritual dimension. One dimension cannot be separated from the other.

Since the mind is both material

and immaterial and the spirit is completely immaterial, health cannot be objective. It is also subjective, or as Leland Kaiser (1994) would say, it is and/both. It is hard after all these years to think of health as subjective when all our standards and guidelines are objective in data.

A human response may best be understood by an example. Have you ever had something like this happen to you? You hear car wheels screeching, and then a thud. You think, where are the kids, and you run to the front door. Before you get there, your heart is racing, you are perspiring, and experiencing an ache in your chest. Most nurses would recognize these symptoms and know each could be explained at a physiological level, by the adrenaline rush. Are these physical symptoms a sign of a medical problem needing a physical treatment such as a medication or an IV?

The event can best be described as a health situation, not a medical situation. This person is experiencing a human response called fear. The physical symptoms are objective, but subjective in cause due to their emergence from the integrated physical, psychological, sociocultural, and spiritual core of the individual. Understanding and knowledge of the body alone does not give one understanding and knowledge of the mind and spirit.

We have concentrated so long on the material or physical component of man that concentrating on the non-material seems uncomfortable. The nonphysical has been disconnected from the description of health. The powerful mind which is both physical and nonphysical provides a natural bridge to the invisible, intangible spirit or will of the person. Yet, it is foreign in our present system to see the person in their connected, inseparable wholeness. The reality is that a strong, healthy heart does not, in itself, make a person healthy. Caring about the health of this society means caring about the people in their wholeness.

I was having lunch one day with

a nurse in California. I remember thinking she was so healthy. Her mind and spirit were vibrant. Yet, she had advanced multiple sclerosis. In the medical care paradigm, "absence of disease," she is not healthy. But in a health paradigm that focuses on the balance of body, mind, and spirit, she is very healthy.

Life events are not medical events. Every person is born and will die. Numerous events will happen throughout the life span. Each day one deals with many different events while trying to maintain the harmony of body, mind, and spirit. Each person owns his/her health. No one has power over another's body, mind or spirit. There are times one needs help and seeks a professional for assistance.

A healthy relationship is one of partnership, not boss-subordinate. The partnership centers on the mission, a mission to achieve the highest level of harmony in body, mind, and spirit. Health is not an episodic, curable, one time thing. Health is a continuous process from birth to death.

Wisdom From The Field

Clinical Scenario: A middle-aged nurse colleague was admitted to the hospital because of complications following an elective surgery. The physician entered the room and said to her, "Martha, I have all your lab tests back and everything is normal. I cannot pinpoint anything that gives insight into any problems." She said to him in a very serious voice, "Sit down. If we are going to be partners and work together on my health, you need to listen to me. I do not care that the lab tests are normal, there must be others that can be taken. *Do you understand that I am very sick. I have a sense of impending doom!*" Those words are piercing to an experienced nurse. They are a concerting symptom from her wholeness. Martha was dead of an unsuspected complication in less than 24 hours.

Her legacy is a clear, poignant message for each of us. We must be in partnership with the people we are privileged to serve. The part we are looking at may appear to be OK, but that does not mean everything is all right. We have to see them in their wholeness, not just a specific body part or their physical status. As health care providers, we began to see the person's problems only as they are related to a specific diagnosis, or within our own specialty. Her concern, unrest, her awareness of her changing physical status, came from her mind and spirit.

What does it mean to care for a person in his/her wholeness? It means consciously seeking the person's story, not just the physical story, but the psychological, sociocultural, and spiritual aspects of the story. It is in the person's story that the uniqueness comes alive and we can learn more about the potential for health. It is not our role to judge the balance, but to support it with maintenance and/or restoration. If we support one domain and not the other, does it matter?

Clinical Scenario: Joann came to the hospital to find out what was causing her severe headaches. She was admitted by a neurologist to whom she had been referred. The nurse caring for her practiced within the new paradigms. He knew the difference between medical care and health care. His mission as a nurse is to optimize a person's health. He understood what that meant. As a result, he sought out the woman's story, not just the physical story.

One evening after report he walked into the room to find Joann and her husband crying. They had been married for 42 years and she considered him her best friend. The nurse discovered that she was crying because she was upset with the new treatment plan. The physician reported to her that he found no reason to explain her headaches and felt it would be best for her to go through some stress and psychological testing. She was filling in some of the psychological forms at the time of the event. Joann said, "I am having headaches and now people think I am nuts, making this up!"

The nurse knew Joann's story,

not just her physical, but psychological, sociocultural, and spiritual story, a natural behavior of the nurse's practice paradigm. He learned that Joann was in love with life and had a wonderful relationship with her husband and children. She was active in the community.

The nurse said that as he listened to Joann's story, he could recognize the balance in her life. The nurse noted that up until the headaches began, Joann's physical status had been very good. Based on her story, the nurse said, "You can lay this questionnaire aside. You have headaches and there is a reason. You are not nuts." The sad part of the story, this nurse stated, took place days later. The nurse entered the room and the woman almost seemed relieved. She was diagnosed with a large ovarian tumor which was malignant. Her only symptom was headaches. She said to the nurse, "At least I am not nuts!"

What can be learned from this story? We all have become specialized. We are specialized in pediatrics, adults,

obstetrics, neurology, oncology, geron-
tology, cardiology, critical care, extended care, home care, and so forth.
We have specialized within the medical
model. Our specialties are within the
physical domain. We actually began to
see the people we serve as hearts, lungs,
nerve cells, body parts, or specific
events.

There is nothing wrong with
specializing, it makes sense. There is so
much to learn, one person cannot learn
it all. It simply should not be done at
the expense or exclusion of the other
domains. If we function out of a medical paradigm as opposed to a health
paradigm, we will continue to see only
part of the picture and mostly see within
our specialty glasses. We will only see
some parts of the body, mind or spirit.
When we see health as medical, or
physical status, broken down into parts,
we cannot impact the health of the
whole person, and in some cases, not
even his/her body.

The new health paradigm
parallels with the principles of Quantum

physics which unfolded the connectiveness of the visible and invisible universe. This paradigm gives us a different set, a more expanded set of guidelines and boundaries. The health paradigm is synchronized with the new paradigm of professional nursing. Albert Einstein (1993) said, "We must build spiritual and scientific bridges linking the nations of the world." In a parallel manner, so must a nurse build spiritual and technological bridges for the health of mankind.

FURTHER EXPLORATION
OF LANDSCAPE

"The best and most beautiful things in the world cannot be seen or even touched. They must be felt with the heart."
- Helen Keller

$\mathcal{T}$he present medical care culture is sensitized and focused on illness. Technological advances poke and prod the physical domain and send forth endless data to analyze, research, and discuss. After a while nurses, especially in the hospital setting, where the majority practice, began to see people only in their physical state. In fact, we used to talk about the people we cared for as the heart in room six, the lung in room nine, and the kidney in room fifteen.

We often didn't refer to the people by name. It makes me think back to what Fox said about the name of the person being the hieroglyph of the soul. We referred to the people we cared for by body parts, not their name. The way we referred to the people was reflective of the paradigm of our practice. The soul or spirit was not as important as the physical care.

The only reinforced data were the materialistic, the physical data. The only reinforced nursing services were those related to the tasks that supported the physical status. Data related to the less tangible aspects of health, that is mind and spirit, were not valued as much by the health care team.

The medical model centers around the weakest, most vulnerable dimension of a human, the body. That is also why the medical model is so important. It is good that we strengthen our weakest link, but it should never be at the expense of the other dimensions or disconnected from them.

In our enthusiasm to provide the

best physical tabernacle for the mind and spirit, we lost sight of the wholeness of the person. *We have watched people live, but not be healthy.* In contrast, many nurses have had the privilege of establishing a relationship with someone who was dying and been in awe of their impressive strength, impressive health, true peace, and harmony of body, mind, and spirit. In a medical care paradigm, if a body fails, it appears we have failed. In a health care paradigm, the time of death may unfold some of our best work. If life is sacred, all components of life are sacred. In wholeness, we tap the spirit, that part of a person that helps one soar above or beyond any physical disability.

Do you believe nursing is a profession? I have asked that question to thousands of our colleagues and they will spontaneously say, "Yes." What does it really mean to be a professional? It means a nurse provides a unique service different from any other professional, different from a doctor, different from an accountant, different from a lawyer. Wouldn't it seem reasonable that nurses, as well as every member of society would know what unique services nurses provide? Do they? Let's put that in perspective.

Are there people in your own immediate family who do not know what you do? Again, thousands of our peers have answered that question with, "Yes." Further evidence of that reality was verified in a study taken across this country by Peter Hart in 1990.

The study had good news and bad news. The good news: Nurses were found to be one of the most respected health care providers in the United States. The bad news makes the good news seem illogical. The bad news: **The general public does not know what we do.** Hart recommended that efforts should be directed toward educating the public on the role and scope of responsibilities of nurses in the health care system.

The confusion in society about what nurses do rests with the confusion of the profession. There are two factors

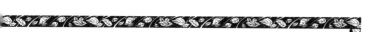

that impact the confusion. One rests with the reality that the majority of all nurses in the United States, as this is written, still practice in the hospital setting. The hospital setting was designed to support medicine and nursing took on the behaviors of the dominant paradigm. The second factor is the inability to decide the education level necessary to practice as a registered nurse. In addition, some nursing education programs continue to focus on the medical and institutional paradigms.

According to Maloney (1992), there are two major characteristics of a professional. One is that professionals have considerable technical expertise. Nurses have considerable technical expertise. The second characteristic: a professional always holds true to the norms of the profession, rather than to those of the organization. Does the second characteristic of a professional make you uncomfortable?

Professional nursing is very different from institutional nursing. See

Figure 4, page 41. Institutional nursing became the norm in the hospital setting. There are very clear reasons for that reality. Nursing has an unusual history. We go to school to learn one profession, but practice in a clinical setting that supports another. The result is frustration. The most common reason nurses give to explain their frustrations is that they "Do not have time to nurse." What does, "We do not have time" mean? If we do not have time to nurse, who will? What would help us practice in the paradigm of professional nursing?

FOLLOWING ANOTHER'S PATH

"Your life is conditioned by your own thoughts, not the thoughts of anyone else."
- Emmet Fox

$\mathcal{P}$hysicians, as nurses, are a committed, intelligent group of prof-essionals devoted to improving the health of humanity. Physicians are one of many health care providers who chose to dedicate their lives to health care. They have been successful in their specific accountability. Because they chose to focus on the body to carry out their mission, does not mean they are not committed to the health paradigm of body, mind, and spirit in balance. Physicians simply chose to master one component. They wisely established educational support and a medical model which guided them in the development of their practice. The success and advancement of their work is evident everywhere.

Nurses work side by side with physicians, physical therapists, psychologists, medicine men, chaplains, dietitians, social workers, etc., all equally committed heath care providers. Nursing plays a significant role in the care of people, not just in the hospitals, but in homes, extended care facilities, schools, clinics, churches, or simply wherever care is needed.

The essence of nursing does not vary depending on the site in which the nurse practices. The wisdom from the field used throughout this writing is often from the hospital setting because it is the most familiar to nurses and the public. It is the place where the majority of nurses still practice. It is also the place where institutional nursing was born and went on to influence the evolution of nursing and health care as we know it today.

Nurses do not go to nursing

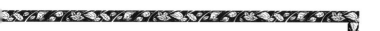

school to become doctors or be like doctors. They did not choose to have primary accountability to diagnose and treat disease, but rather to diagnose and treat the human response. One is not more important than the other; it is simply a different choice. The work of supporting humanity in its health requires many different types of professionals. It may be said one day that the work of every human is to be a health care provider, working in one way or another to maintain, restore, or improve the health of humanity.

Whether one chooses to be in the work of accounting, water and plumbing, law, sanitation, food services, transportation, politics, education, operations, or research, the work is about health. And it may be said that the hope for a healthy humanity will rest in the ability of each professional to work together in partnerships focused on the mission of health. Is that what the present chaos is all about?

With many health care providers, a pattern of relating to one another emerged. Relationships began to mimic the health care organizational systems and structures. Three of the most well known bureaucratic and hierarchical cultures are church, military, and hospitals. The bureaucratic, hierarchical culture is one of power, we-they, boss-subordinate, and "I am more important than you." It is not about partnership. Because of the importance of the system's culture and structures on relationships, the next book in this series will be dedicated to the foundational issue of partnership.

The bureaucratic culture led to the health care paradigm being weakened. Instead of a focus on body, mind, and spirit in balance, it became one characterized by the body being more important than mind and spirit, doctor more than nurse, and manager more important than staff. It was a predictable evolution based on history and the nature of usual patterns of human relationships. It is simply an old paradigm.

The face of nursing changed with

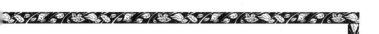

the fast paced evolution of medicine. The professional image became closely linked with the nursing practice within the hospital setting. Institutional nursing as previously mentioned became the norm. The health care paradigm and professional nursing were lost in the enthusiasm for the medical paradigm. It has only been in the closing of the last decade of this millennium that the society awakened to its need for a health care system, and a less costly medical care system. We are all living the inevitable chaos that comes with the breaking of old patterns of thinking.

Nurses have a unique wisdom that comes from their relationship with the people needing care. The nurse today spends more time with people needing health care than any other provider. They are present during birthing and birth, in schools, work settings, churches, camps, extended care settings, homes, on battle fields, and at the bedside of those dying.

In the hospital, the nurse is the

only continuous provider for the person receiving care. The other health care providers; including doctor, dietitian, chaplain, physical therapist, social worker, and others, come and go. The other providers are episodic. The only reason a person is hospitalized today is that they need continuous nursing care. Wouldn't you think if you wanted to see the most impeccable place to practice nursing, it would be in the hospital?

Nursing practice has been impacted by the medical care paradigm and has played a major role in the development of quality medical care. Nursing has great accountability to lead the society out of the present chaos, not just because they are the largest group of health care providers in the world, but because of the day to day realities of the present health care system and the connections of nurses in a very unique way to the people of this society. However, we cannot lead the society from a medical care to a health care system unless we know and believe in it ourselves.

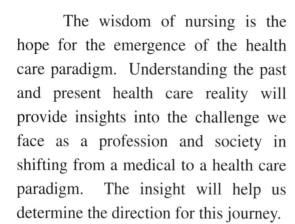

The wisdom of nursing is the hope for the emergence of the health care paradigm. Understanding the past and present health care reality will provide insights into the challenge we face as a profession and society in shifting from a medical to a health care paradigm. The insight will help us determine the direction for this journey.

CONSIDERING A DIFFERENT
ROUTE, DIFFERENT DIRECTION

*"The greatest battles of life are fought out
every day in the chambers of our hearts."*
- McKay

*A*t what point did we begin to lose sight of nursing's unique role in the achievement of health, that is, body, mind, and spirit in balance, in harmony? Over 100 years ago Florence Nightingale warned us about the need for vigilance in our thinking about our role. She reminded us of that role when she said, "The role of the nurse is to put the patient in the best possible condition for nature to restore, or maintain health, prevent or cure disease and illness." She knew health was more than preventing or curing disease. She saw nursing as having accountability for health, which is of course, inclusive of the physical status.

Over 100 years ago Florence expressed concern about what was happening with nursing practice in the hospital. She said, "The world, more especially the hospital world, is in such a hurry, is moving so fast, that it is too easy to slide into bad habits before we are aware." It is amazing that she spoke those words so long ago. It is as if they were spoken for today. Institutional nursing, the dependent task-dominated practice where nursing services became directed by doctors' orders and hospital policies and procedures, is the bad habit we fell into.

The tasks are not the problem. The problem is the mind set, the mind set that the task ordered by the physician, is nursing. Florence recognized where the problem was coming from and she said, "Medicine and nursing must never be mixed up...it spoils both." We mixed them up. Nursing lost sight of nursing and medicine began to see only the body. The mind and spirit became subordinate. The concept of health was pushed into the background.

Nursing took on the characteristics of the setting. During a period of time in the 1900's nursing began to see its practice differently. Our work centered and connected with the body, more than the mind and spirit. DePree (1992) shared a quote by Antoine de Saint Exupery, that said, "It is only with the heart that one can see right, what is essential is invisible to the eye." We lost sight of the invisible mind and spirit, the scale tipped, and the concept of balance was lost.

Ironically, Florence also gave some advice about how to offset the shift and how to remain clear. She said, "What is our needful thing, to have high principles at the bottom of all without having laid our foundation, there is small use in building up our details."

Physicians were very clear about the principles of their practice and created a structure to support them. Did

Florence recognize there was no structure, no foundation within the culture to support the beliefs of nursing? Did she recognize there was no clarity amongst her nursing colleagues on what was most important within the realm of nursing? Did she understand the power of the structure and systems design of the hospital setting and the impact on practice? Did nursing create a foundation, but it got lost? Was there a foundation that supported both nursing and medicine, but not partnership? Was nursing not clear enough or strong enough to establish a foundation to help develop the profession? Was society not interested?

Florence suggested that before we could prevent mixing up medicine and nursing, we must be clear on what nursing is, what it is about. Clarity on the essence of nursing is the foundation. Before nurses and physicians can partner on their accountabilities to health, each must be clear about their practice and service. Each need to clarify the principles, the core beliefs of his/her professional accountability.

Covey (1990) notes that "Once we become relatively independent, our challenge is to become effectively interdependent with others." Physicians were clear. Nursing was not clear. Instead of the merging of nursing and medical practices in partnership, medicine became dominant and the foundational piece necessary to support nursing was not established in the hospital setting. It has taken a century for the impact of that historical reality to be felt.

In the middle of the twentieth century it became cheaper to give large numbers of people care in hospitals rather than in homes. Instead of nurses coming to the hospital setting and establishing a foundation to support the essence of nursing practice, the practice evolved around the policies, procedures, rituals, patterns, and routines supporting the practice of medicine.

The number of hospitals began to increase and the number of nurses necessary to care for the people in the hospitals began to increase. The hospital became the center of the health care system. The medical model, "absence of disease," became the foundation. There was no foundation within the health care system built on the integration of physical, psychological, sociocultural, and spiritual domain.

The work of establishing the foundation is still to be done. The success of that effort rests first with the ability of nurses to collectively be clear on the essence of their profession. Not just clear at a theoretical level, but clear at the day to day practice level. Secondarily, it rests with the willingness to do the work of establishing the foundation in the clinical settings.

Over the last twelve years, a growing group of thousands of nurses practicing daily in rural, community, and university hospital settings have committed to the work of implementing a foundation. See Appendix, pages 167-169, for a listing. It is the learnings from their efforts, along with others, that will be shared throughout this series. These nurses are linked through the Clinical Practice Model (CPM) Resource Center whose mission is: To enhance partnering relationships and world linkages for the generation of collective knowledge and wisdom that will continually improve the structure, process, and outcomes of professional nursing and community health care services.

FOUNDATION STEPPING STONES

Florence noted that the practice foundation must be based on principles. Just as our personal belief systems guide us in our day to day actions and decisions, nursing core beliefs are necessary to guide us in our practice. What is the foundation, the principles or the core beliefs about the essence of nursing? If there are core beliefs, would they not be the same and evident in the actions of all nurses, regardless of where they are practicing? If core beliefs are important, would not each nurse be able to talk about them and demonstrate how

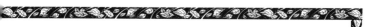

they are lived in practice?

The power of paradigms can best be realized when talking with thousands of nurses who practice in the hospital setting built within a medical and institutional culture. The outcomes of the two patterns of thinking are most evident in the difficulty of the bedside practitioners to: first, define clearly their unique scope of service, and second, live consistently what they believe is the essence of nursing in their practice fields.

DECIDING THE ROUTE,
THE DIRECTION

"And still, cure without care is as dehumanizing as a gift given with a cold heart. But cure without care makes us into rulers, controllers, manipulators, and prevents a real community from taking shape. Cure without care can be offending instead of liberating."
- Henri Nouwen

*T*here should be no nurse unclear on the essence of nursing, the mission of nursing, and the role and scope of professional accountabilities. Somehow we must overcome the limits of language, and the inability to articulate to every person the essence of our profession. It is not enough to say nurses care. Most humans care. Nurses do not care more than physicians, more than other providers, more than the mother of the child needing our services, the spouse or significant others. The way in which we care is determined by the role we consciously chose. The nurse must be clear on that role and its driving beliefs. We demonstrate caring by practicing excellence within our role.

The professional beliefs, the foundation, the essence of nursing should not vary from setting to setting, nurse to nurse, shift to shift, city to city. Core beliefs are like the principles of nature. For example, the plant is governed by laws of nature. A person can choose not to water a plant, but it will die. It is governed by something of a higher nature than the person's individual understanding or agreement. Stephen Covey (1990) noted that principles are like the laws of nature. They are a compass. They give direction when there is no path or map. Core beliefs provide a compass for nurses as they carry out their role daily. *The core beliefs are the compass for this journey.*

Goethe, the German philosopher, summed up well the need for core beliefs when he said, "Things that matter most should never be at the mercy of things which matter least." Nurse, what matters most? We have learned from our past that if we collectively are uncertain, it is easy to lose sight of what we believe, especially in a culture that has no systems or structures to support it. It is easy to lose sight of beliefs during fast paced change, especially if they are not written on the soul.

Over the last twenty years a process was begun to not only seek out clarity on the beliefs about the essence of nursing, but also, take on the work of living them. I have surveyed, formally and informally, thousands of colleagues from student to novice to expert. What has become apparent is the ease to which nurses can agree on core beliefs. The difficulty is how to say them in simple terms that mean the same on paper as they do in the heart. *This precedes the ultimate challenge, to live them.*

I have shared the evolving core beliefs with thousands across the United States and Canada. During the discussion and dialogue surrounding the core beliefs, a common ground on nursing unfolds. One colleague said, "How could you not believe in them, they are like America, apple pie, and Chevrolet." However, when asked, "Do you live them," the answer is most consistently, "No." Our peers then proceed to say things, such as, "I can't in the setting in which I practice," "If you knew what my unit was like, you would understand why I cannot live them," "There is no place for us to go to practice what we believe." This incongruency needs to change.

The incongruency between what we believe and our inability to live our beliefs needs to change. Some ways to help that happen is the subject of another book. The direction for the rest of this journey will become clear as we explore each of the core beliefs.

SIMPLIFYING THE DIRECTIONS

The core beliefs are the work of thousands of bedside practitioners who took on the effort to clarify and articulate the beliefs about the essence of health and the essence of nursing. In addition, these many nurses have made a choice to lead the work of creating an environment that supports living them.

See Figure 5 for the present wording of the core beliefs. Recently the core beliefs were reviewed by hundreds of nurse colleagues, as well as many people we care for, their significant others, members of hospital boards of trustees, people in the community, physicians, other health care team members, and administrators in 19 states and Canada. The strong message from the reviewing process was a call to simplify the wording of the core beliefs. The purpose of the review was to help us clarify what we personally believe about health care and nursing.

A lesson learned over the twelve years from the review of core beliefs is

FIGURE 5

CORE BELIEFS

- ♥ Quality emerges from an environment driven by mission, principles and partnerships.

- ♥ Each person has the right to receive care that optimizes health which is body, mind, and spirit in balance.

- ♥ Each person is accountable to explain and provide his/her unique contribution to care.

- ♥ Health care is coordinated and delivered in partnership with the person receiving care.

- ♥ New ways of thinking are essential to continually improve health care throughout the life span.

- ♥ Empowerment begins with each person and is enhanced by relationships and systems design.

the importance of the process of the review. It is the dialogue and discussion with one another about our beliefs that helps each person become clearer in his/her own mind. It is that process that facilitates each person imprinting the core beliefs on the soul. This journey is an opportunity for you to review the stated core beliefs. You may have different words, different ideas that speak to your heart, jot them down. It could be a great learning for many if you would be willing to share them. The Appendix, page 167-169, directs how to share your thoughts.

One core belief does not build on the other. Each speaks to the indivisible whole of our practice. The stories, the wisdom from the field, will guide us in the exploration of core beliefs. The core beliefs are clearer when discussed in relation to the mission of nursing, and focused on the people we are privileged to serve. The mission and the core beliefs are the magnet of the compass.

CONSTRUCTING NEW ROADS -
LAYING GRAVEL

"Principles are self-evident, self-validating natural laws. They don't change or shift. They provide "true north" direction to our lives when navigating the "streams" of our environment."
                                    - Stephen Covey

Core Belief: **Quality emerges from an environment driven by mission, principles, and partnerships.**

*H*ave you ever heard someone in the practice setting say something like the following? "You just can't give good care around here; there is too much red tape, policies, procedures, and bureaucracy!" "This organization doesn't support patient care, only bottom line...etc." "They just don't care about patients or the people that work here." "They, they they........." Do you believe the environment, or the culture of the practice setting impacts the person's care?

We are the culture. We are the organization. We are they. We are the environment. We create it, not someone else. *What the nurses and other health care givers collectively believe, will be the greatest factor determining the type of culture that surrounds them.* Nurses are the largest number of professional health care providers in the world. A health care environment, and the hope for that environment, sits in our hands. What type of environment do we believe is necessary for quality to emerge?

Mission

Do you believe quality emerges from an environment driven by mission? Mission, along with the core beliefs, is the perfect place to begin. It is foundational, the gravel bed. It is about purpose and the meaning of life. It is about the reason a person or an organization exists. Are you clear on your personal mission? What gives you purpose and meaning in your life? If you have not written your mission down or are uncertain of it, you may be putting yourself and others at risk. It would be good to stop right here, before this journey goes any further, and write down your personal mission. Underwood (1993) captured the importance of mission from her Native American ancestors who said, "That the people explained to one another that Purpose may be better than Finding."

When I added nurse to my name, I became accountable to the mission of nursing. Everyone has the right to hold me accountable to it. It is no different than when one adds the role of mother, father, lawyer, or physician to their name. All of us will be held accountable to the mission of the role we chose. The mission of nursing is to optimize each person's health, that is, body, mind, and spirit in balance. It calls for great knowledge, commitment, and expertise. Here is an important question: **Is your personal mission and the mission of nursing in synch?** If not, for your own health, the health of the people you serve, and the people you practice with, *please address this issue.*

Have you ever come to work, looked to see who will be on the team with you and find yourself saying something like this. "Oh darn, Mary is on tonight!" You go down the hall, run into another colleague and say, "Did you see, Mary is on tonight?" The other person says, "Oh no, not Mary!" Of course no one says anything to Mary. No one works well with Mary. Mary does her own thing. In fact, no one holds Mary accountable to the mission of nursing. There is confusion between personal issues and mission. If the team is not synchronized in its commitment to the mission, it is not good for anyone.

If the unit, setting or organization is driven by the mission to optimize the health of communities (and most say they are), all decisions and service will be based on what is best to optimize the health of the people they serve. The service, and the decisions, will not be driven by the desire to be number one, have the largest market, do more surgeries, or have the best bottom line in the community. That may in fact be the result of living their mission, but it is not the mission. If either the individuals or the professionals who make up the organization do not have a synchronized mission, quality will not emerge.

Principles

Do you believe quality emerges from an environment driven by principles? The words quality care are heard often. Everybody is talking about quality care. The 1980's was the era of quality. Unless one is living in a closet, he/she knows of the CQI, TQM, QI/QA programs that are taking place in every business setting. Some think of it as a buzz word; it is not. Some will say, "We support quality, but it is a hard thing to define." No, it is not. Do you personally know when you have received quality service? There are principles of quality that should be shaping the environment. They are not a secret. There are three critical characteristics of quality service. One, the providers must be competent in their services. Two, the services must be integrated within the team. And three, the services must match the health needs of the individual they serve.

The three characteristics emerge from the principles of quality. Donabedian (1980, 1982) has studied and written about the following characteristics of quality health care services. He noted quality care reflects the principles of coordination and, mutually determined, individualized service which has no duplication, replication throughout the delivery.

Clinical Question: Do you think there is a nurse caring for a person who does not know the person's story? Do you think nurses know the physical story, but little about the mind or spirit? Do you think there is a nurse who has not established mutuality with the person? Do you think that at this moment there are nurses asking a question that has been asked previously by another health care provider? Is there clarity about what questions are appropriate to be *reasked* the person such as, "Do you have any new concerns?"

Do you think there is a nurse who knows important information about the uniqueness of a person, but the physical therapist caring for the same person does not know it? Do you believe at this moment there is a nurse charting something in one place that had already been charted in another? That is duplication and replication. This is not quality care. If the principles of quality are not at the roots of every provider's service, quality will not emerge. Principles of quality link the mission and partnerships.

Partnership

Do you believe quality emerges in an environment of partnership? The mission is the heartbeat, but it cannot be achieved without forming partnerships between the people we serve and the other interdisciplinary team members. Partnership is the joining of hearts, hands, and minds of at least two people with a common mission driven by clarity on what matters most in the relationship. Do you think the relationship that the nurse has with the person seeking health care will impact the person's healing process? Do you think the person receiving care can tell if one provider has a good relationship with the other providers? Do you think this impacts their healing process? Partnerships are pivotal to the emergence of quality.

Wisdom From The Field

Living the core beliefs can be difficult. The rituals, patterns, and routines of institutional practice have become the norms. One ritual and pattern that is common and violates this core belief is **visiting hours.** Visiting hours interfere with the mission, partnerships, and principles. Here are two situations that demonstrate this point and were shared by people we cared for.

Clinical Scenario One: A mother of a 17 year old child who had been a victim of a car accident was not allowed to stay at his side. She said to us: "Who do you think you are? Who do you think you are to tell me what is best for my child? I gave life to him, raised him, and loved him for 17 years and you actually think you know what is best for him. You even think you know what is best for me and you don't even know me! You care for him a short while; I will care for him the rest of his life. Who do you think you are?" She shared this information months after the accident and the emotion in her voice was as if it had happened that day. What does this say about our mission, principles, and partnerships?

Clinical Scenario Two: An 80 year old fragile woman who came to the hospital with her very ill husband said, "I don't understand. I have lived with and loved John for 60 years. We have shared everything, the good times and the bad, but always we were together. It seems reasonable that I should be with him in his death. I do not take up much room, but the ICU nurse said I would have to wait for visiting hours."

Who do we think we are? Visiting hours is just *one* example of the rituals, policies, and routines that have driven our actions. It is a strong institutional practice pattern. Somehow in all of this history, we actually came to think that it was our right to be at the side of the person needing care and everyone else, including their own family, was a visitor. You might be thinking, I would never have separated the woman from her husband, John. It doesn't matter what you would have done. *It matters that any one of us would have done it.* We are all connected. When there is a lack of clarity on what we believe is important, these types of situations will continue over and over again.

CONSTRUCTING NEW ROADS - LAYING CEMENT

"Hope sees the invisible, feels the intangible and achieves the impossible."
- unknown

Core Belief: **Each person has the right to receive care that optimizes health which is body, mind and spirit in balance.**

*T*his core belief speaks about the heart of nursing. It says that regardless of age, race, status, education, sexual orientation, social, economic or political status, and so forth, each person has the right to receive care. It also speaks to the desired outcomes of that care. It says that whenever a nurse or any other provider is present, the person can count on his/her health being optimized. It does not say only their medical status, but their health status as well.

No matter what the situation is, this core belief says the nurse will bring light and hope that optimizes the person's health. Do you believe this? Remember, hope does not mean false hope, such as to say they will live when they are dying. Hope is the assurance that the best possible situation will be created for this person's ultimate health, the best situation, not just for their body, but their mind and spirit. Health is not just an event, it is the state of being. For some people, their optimal health may be death. Nursing is not limited by any situation from birth to death. The opportunities to impact the health of a person are unlimited in this core belief.

This core belief calls for different patterns of thinking and action other than those imbedded within the medical and institutional paradigms. What does it really mean to be rooted in a health paradigm which is inclusive of body,

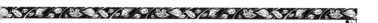

mind, and spirit? It helps one see that nursing is a profession of science and art. It exemplifies the definition of nursing given by Sister Simone Roach (1991) who said, "Nursing is the professionalization of the human capacity to care through the acquisition and supplication of knowledge, attitudes, and skills required for nursing's prescribed roles." It requires great intelligence and expertise, not just in the matters of body, but in mind and spirit. It calls for a different kind of thinking, different types of inquiry and different types of action.

Wisdom From The Field

Clinical Scenario: Jack was a 38 year old man who was rushed to the emergency department with severe, crushing chest pain. He was awake, talking, and in great distress. Shortly after his arrival, he arrested. He was intubated and resuscitated with CPR and given medications. Something very unusual happened. He became conscious and aware during cardiac massage. However, if the massage was stopped he would lose consciousness and arrest.

Jack's EKG showed a massive heart attack and the cardiologist proclaimed there was no way for this man to survive with the present technology. The nurse thought about his health: his body, mind, and spirit, not just his failing body. His spirit would be leaving it soon. What would give him balance, harmony at this time? What about his story? Who was he in his wholeness? He was a husband, father, and brother.

What could be done to make this the best possible situation for him at this time? What does harmony and balance mean during imminent death? He was able to communicate and was mouthing words. His wife was brought to the bedside, not an accepted practice in this setting at that time. She was told of the situation and was brought to be with him and speak with him. The nurse wondered, was there anything special on his mind? Her inquiry resulted in a

"Yes." He needed to see his son who was eight years old and presently playing at his little league game. The son and father had a disagreement earlier in the day. They continued cardiac massage until his son was brought to his bedside and he was able to mouth "I love you" to him, as well as his wife and his brother. Resuscitation was eventually stopped and his spirit left his body.

What is this health paradigm all about anyway? It is related to the lessons learned from Quantum physics. Everything is connected. There is a dynamic connection not only between body, mind, and spirit, but from one person to another. Within a medical care paradigm, we became attuned to health as body, one person's body, the person being cared for. What is the accountability when there is no more that can be done for the body?

A health model is not focused on just the body. It is focused on the *connection* of body, mind, and spirit. It is this reality that changes practice in so many ways. In a health paradigm, we will never just care for one body, but the whole person. We will care for their significant others with whom they connect in mind and spirit. To care for this gentleman, we need to care for those he loves, those who will live on after he is gone. His family is a part of his health and a part of the health of our communities. Health is not just about the failing of one body.

Does this type of care matter? The next night after Jack died, the nurse noted a man sitting patiently by the entrance in the emergency department. It was a very busy night and some people had been waiting for hours. Several critically ill patients had arrived and two people with burns were transferred out. Things finally calmed down. When approached, the man said he was the brother of the man who died yesterday, and he came to thank the nurses. He felt that the decision to have his brother's wife, son, and family be with him was invaluable and helped them in their grief. It was so important, he said, that he would be willing to wait for hours to say, "Thank you."

Although we are novices in the health paradigm, it is the hope for the future of our humanity. Does each person have the right to expect nurses to practice from a health paradigm?

CONSTRUCTING NEW ROADS - THE BUSINESS LOOP

"Our deeds are like stones cast into the pool of time; though they themselves may disappear, their ripples extend to eternity."

- Unknown

Core Belief: **Each person is accountable to explain and provide his/her unique contribution to care.**

$\mathcal{T}$he previous core belief said each person has the right to receive nursing care and that the nursing service should contribute to the person's health status. What are we saying differently here? Do you believe the nurse, as well as every other provider, should know how to explain and provide their unique

service? For this to be achieved, providers have to: first, be as clear as possible on their unique service, then be aware of every other provider's service to help the person understand the unique contribution of each.

It is not appropriate for any nurse or any other provider to be uncertain as to what nurses do, especially during the chaos that is happening in the health care arena. The top "C", cost, is controlling most decisions being made to redesign, re-engineer, regenerate, and to reconfigure the health care system. The first and more obvious way to cut cost is by decreasing the number of people providing care. Nurses are the largest group of providers in the world; therefore, cut nurses, cut cost. If one is uncertain as to what nurses do, cutting them is easier. If people think nursing is only institutional in nature, it makes sense to cut nurses. Why?

There is not a task that is done by the nurse that can't be done equally as well by a nonprofessional taken off the street and taught in less than two weeks.

Thousands of people every day in their homes and their work settings do many of the tasks nurses do. For example, millions of people take their own meds every day. People are doing their own peritoneal dialysis, hemodialysis, TPN therapy, and antibiotic therapy.

Significant others are doing extensive open wound care which may be more safely treated in the home because of the risk of nosocomial infection in the hospital. Significant others are doing complex respiratory care with ventilator dependent people. Medical treatments such as cardiotonic drugs and chemotherapy are being administered in the home. **Nurse, what is it you do that is so important, that when you are not there, it matters? Do you know?**

A great deal has been learned over the last twelve years of working together with nurses across this country and Canada to create practice environments that support living the core beliefs. The importance of this core belief, that states we must be clear about

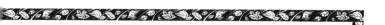

our service, has been directly linked with the success of transition from old to new ways of thinking and practice. Action cannot be taken to create a supportive environment to help nurses provide their unique service, if there is uncertainty over what the services actually are.

The first step in clarifying our service is to find a practical way to define the unique professional services nurses provide. This society expects each professional to be able to articulate and provide their unique services. The norm of institutional nursing has confused nursing as well as the public. That is why Hart (1990) suggested educating the public on the role and scope of nursing. That is also why this will be the longest segment written for all of the core beliefs.

Nursing care was defined within a service driven framework that parallels with society's expectations. There are three categories of service one can expect from a nurse (Wesorick, 1990). They are listed in Figure 6 as delegated,

FIGURE 6

Nursing's Unique Professional Services:

Delegated

Services which enhance the
health of a person and require a
physician's order.

Interdependent

Services which enhance health by
assessing, monitoring,
detecting, and preventing
physiological complications
associated with certain health
situations or treatment plans.

Independent

Services which enhance health
by assessing, monitoring,
detecting, diagnosing, and treating
the human responses to health
status or situation.

interdependent, and independent. Each of the three services will be discussed within the framework of clinical situations to clarify the depth of the category in a practical sense. The three professional services are very different from institutional nursing services.

The practice norms for institutional and professional services are very different. The learnings, from nurses practicing in 30 different settings in 19 different states and Canada, have shown that there is great inconsistency in the delivery of the three services. However, there is a pattern. There is a greater consistency in delegated, less in interdependent, and little consistency in the independent services. This work has taught us that one of the greatest challenges we have as nurses is **to know nursing as well as we know medicine, and have the public know nursing as well as they know medicine.**

Wisdom From The Field

Clinical Scenario: The nurses caring for Matt had transitioned from a medical to a health model, from institutional to professional nursing, and to a practice driven by the core beliefs. Matt was an 18 year old young gentleman whose dream was to represent his country at the Olympics. He was well on his way to realizing that dream. He had many victories, many medals, many trophies, and held the state record in his running field. One day while Matt was out running, he was hit by a car and his life instantly changed. He sustained a cervical fracture and would never walk or run again.

Do you think Matt, his parents, and significant others knew what to expect from the nurses? Do you think they understood nursing's unique services and how they differ from the physician's role in Matt's care? Being clear on the essence of nursing means understanding the services, not just the tasks, a nurse carries out.

The nurse caring for Matt explained nursing's unique services to his mother, Mrs. West, in this way. "Mrs. West, our goal is to help Matt reach his ultimate health." His mother asked if the nurse could make his paralysis go away. "No, we cannot make his paralysis go away." She went on to explain, "His health will be different than before, but he can be healthy." Nurse, do you believe Matt can be healthy? The answer depends on which paradigm drives your practice. She explained, "Matt will need a lot of care and there are three special services the nurses will be providing that you can count on."

Delegated Service

The first category of service is called *delegated.* These are services nurses will provide that require a physician's order. The nurse does not carry these orders out because the physician ordered them; in fact, that would be negligence and the nurse could be liable. The nurse carries them out because it is the right thing for Matt at that time. The administration of the antibiotics that Matt is receiving is an example. The doctor must order it, but before the nurses give it, they will know what organism this antibiotic is effective against, and check the culture, if available, for sensitivity/resistance.

The nurse must know that the drug dose is right for Matt and what the side effects are in order to assess him closely. In fact, it will typically be the nurse who will note if Matt has any side effects and will call the doctor for a change, or additional treatment. This is a high level service requiring great knowledge and critical thinking.

Giving the medication to Matt is a small part of our services. The critical part is the assessment and how it correlates to Matt's status. Anybody can give the drug. In fact, in time, Matt can take his own, but before that happens, the nurse will teach him what he needs to know to do it safely.

Delegated services are professional and very different from

institutional practice. Of the three categories, there is more consistency on this service than the next two. The reason is its close association with the medical model. What mattered in the old paradigm, was getting the medications passed or treatments done on time, and not leaving anything for the next shift. The professional paradigm is very different.

Interdependent Service

There is a second category of service you can expect for Matt. We call it *interdependent.* These are the services which enhance Matt's health by assessing, monitoring, detecting, and preventing physiological complications associated with certain health situations or treatment plans.

Matt was on the ventilator, had a central line, naso-gastric tube, chest tube, foley and was on a special bed. Do these treatments and his diagnosis put him at risk for various complications? It was explained to Mrs. West that each nurse who cares for Matt will know what he is at risk for, know the signs and symptoms of the potential problem, and will assess Matt for them. Nurses will also provide services that will prevent Matt from having complications. These services are not ordered by the physician, they are services nurses provide because they are registered nurses.

Matt's mother, Mrs. West, was informed that the nurse is not the only one who could provide these services; the doctor could as well. However, the physician is at the bedside an average of 5-15 minutes a day. Matt is at risk for these complications 24 hours a day and that is why the presence of the nurse is so critical. As his need for this service decreases, the frequency of the nurses at his bedside will decrease.

Interdependent services are professional and very different from institutional practice. The central line would be a good way to compare the practice patterns. The institutional nurse would know there was a central line, know which IV was running, the rate of the IV, if the lines had been changed, and if it was on time or not.

Professional nursing, regardless of which nurse was accountable for caring for Matt, would additionally know the common complications of the central line, the signs and symptoms of those complications, would have assessed for the complications, and carried out interventions to prevent the complications.

Independent Service

The third category of service is *independent*. This service is closely linked with the reason many chose to become a nurse. These are the services which enhance Matt's health by assessing, monitoring, detecting, diagnosing, and treating his human response. It assures that Matt will never be seen as a heart, lung, kidney, medical diagnosis, DRG, critical path or map. He will be seen as a special young man, who happens to have a cervical fracture and is personally responding to the condition in a certain way. The nurse will help Matt and his significant others through their personal responses.

The national nomenclature for service is nursing diagnosis. This speaks to nursings' primary accountability to diagnose and treat the human response. The response is embedded in the integration of body, mind, and spirit, which is about health, the root of nursing. This category addresses the least tangible, but the most powerful part of our practice. The tangible components of Matt's care, the ventilator, NG, central line, chest tube, and foley, can keep the provider busy and are important to his physiological progression. What about his overall health?

What type of response do you think Matt had to his new reality? The first and most common answer given, not just by nurses, but other health care colleagues, has been anger, followed by denial, depression, disbelief, and grief. Grief is the diagnostic category for the other listed symptoms. Matt, as well as his family, was grieving intensely.

You may be thinking, how big a deal is it to diagnose and treat the human response? It seems so obvious. What makes it obvious? Knowing Matt's story. Diagnosing the human response is very different from diagnosing the medical condition. The human response is personal and the accuracy of diagnosis, as well as treatment, rests with the knowledge of the person's physical, psychological, sociocultural, and spiritual story. A medical diagnosis can be made without the rest of the story. The diagnosis of the human response cannot.

In a culture of institutional nursing, the care would be different. The focus is not on the human response, only on the medical problems. The greatest evidence of this reality is the type of exchange report given from one nurse to the other. It centers around the meds given, the treatments done, and the physiological status. Little information about the person's unique story and human response is integrated into the discussion of care from one colleague to the next.

A good way to understand the difference between institutional and professional practice as it relates to this category of service is by thinking about the following question: Do you have peers who would never consider giving an unfamiliar medication without looking it up? Do you think that some of those same peers have not read a recent article on how to treat the human response of grief? The paradigm that drives a nurse's practice will determine his/her practice pattern.

There are some nurses who diagnose grief, but treat it as their parents taught them. In many cases, the approach is dysfunctional. *There is no policy and procedure for treating the human response.* Life experiences are not enough. A new paradigm calls for new and expanded knowledge, thinking, and expertise. In fact, some of the expertise of the old paradigms interfere with successful transition from institutional to professional nursing.

The human response flows from

the integration of body, mind, and spirit. Do you think nurses have a common ground on the understanding, valuing, and use of the nursing diagnosis process related to the human response? Which of these three: body, mind or spirit, do you believe will play the most significant role in optimizing Matt's health? Thousands of nurses and other health care providers, when asked the same question, were consistent in their response of "Spirit."

How good are you at diagnosing and treating the human response, the integration of body, mind, and spirit? I asked that question of a neurosurgeon and he said, "Not very good." My response to him was, "That is OK. You have chosen to be a neurosurgeon; you need to be a master of neuro-surgery. It is, however, important that you, as a physician, know the critical role his spirit will play, and value the related work as part of his ultimate health. Nurses have primary accountability for that service. Did you know, that is what our formal definition of professional nursing promises?"

He did not know nurses were accountable, I went on to say, "Nurses know the importance of the surgery you do. It is good for you to know what nursing practice is and the impact of it. One service is not more important than the other. They are both essential. That is why a person needs a physician and a nurse in partnership. That is why we are taking on the work to change our practice from institutional to professional nursing."

Matt was lucky. He had a nurse who knew and practiced the full scope of service. She was a role model for the transition from institutional to professional nursing. She studied and learned about the human responses and treatments. And when Matt presented symptoms of anger, her exploration with him helped her differentiate between grief and spiritual distress. He was angry, a common symptom of grief, but, his anger was because he had lost his purpose and meaning in life, running.

Losing one's purpose and

meaning in life is spiritual distress. Matt's nurse held a conference with the whole team to look at what could be done to support Matt throughout his human response. The word lucky may seem crude to you, but it did matter which nurse was at Matt's bedside, and which paradigm was driving the nurse's practice. It was the difference in his outcomes.

Knowing the three categories of professional nursing services and understanding the services related to each is important, but just the beginning. Shifting practice from institutional to professional patterns of care takes a great deal of conscious thinking and work. This core belief clearly states that the nurse is accountable, not just to know, but also to carry out, his/her unique scope of practice.

The following clinical scenario occurred while working with the registered nurses in the emergency department related to their full scope of practice. Discussion about the nurse's unique role in a health care paradigm versus a medical care paradigm and the responsibility for the three categories of service became frustrating.

There had been much discussion and dialogue about the feasibility of the full scope of services in this strong medical model setting, and the ability of the nurse in the short time framework to provide delegated, interdependent, and especially independent services. Could they really be accountable for all three? This core belief says that when there is a nurse present, a person can expect, not part of his/her unique services, but all, if the services are indicated. An exercise was suggested to raise the awareness of the scope of practice. The suggestion was to stand by the bed and ask oneself, "Have I nursed this person?" Then specifically recall the three services, delegated, interdependent, and inde-pendent.

Wisdom From The Field

Clinical Scenario: A nurse working in the emergency room was struggling with how to provide nursing care within the health framework and within the scope of professional nursing practice. She described herself as the institutional queen. However, she said, "I believe in all of the "core beliefs", but don't practice them." She announced one day that she had made a decision that she was going to start living them, not just talk about them. She openly stated to her peers that she didn't know how to live them and would need their help and support.

She was assigned to the trauma section when a seven year old boy named Bill was admitted. He had been a passenger in a car with his mother and sister when they were involved in a multi-vehicle accident. His mother was pronounced dead at the scene, his older sister was unharmed, and he sustained serious injury. The sister knew her mother was dead and she stayed at the side of her brother. No other family were present.

The nurse was comfortable with the sister at the bedside, and let her know they would be working very hard to help her brother. The belief of partnership was her strength. She was very aware that his sister would play an important role in his ultimate health. The nurse recalled thinking in the early stages of care, "I hope he will make it" and remembered thinking she was glad when he started to cry because it was a good sign. His sister went to comfort him and her presence helped calm him.

As Bill stabilized, the nurse asked the secretary to call Ped's ICU for a bed to transfer him. The secretary came back and reported that PICU was full and he would have to stay in the emergency room until they could work something out. The nurse would need to special him until transfer could take place.

Bill began to cry for his mother. The nurse said nothing. He kept crying for his mother. His sister said, "Mom can't come, she is dead." He said he didn't care that she was dead, he needed her. And he cried even more for her. The nurse said she remembered saying to herself, "Oh, I wish he didn't know his mother was dead; what do I do? Boy, I wish we could transfer him. This is why I work in Emergency; we get them through the crisis, we like that type of work, and we send them on. I prefer it that way." During this frustration she recalled the exercise given during the two day workshop, to stand at the foot of the bed and ask, have I nursed him?

She went through each of the categories of professional services and thought to herself, "Delegated, I am impressive. Interdependent, I am equally impressive. Independent, the human response, oh gee, I do not know what to do. His grief is so apparent. I wish I could transfer him." She went out to the desk and sought help. There is a little humor in how it unfolded.

The nurse caring for Bill is a very calm, competent nurse. She is one you would like to have around when there is a crisis. She went out to the station and said in a tense voice, "I need help." Everyone jumped up, one nurse thought that the little boy must be in great trouble because she seemed so tense.

Then she said, "I need help with this human response stuff." Everyone sat right back down. She called in some resources, one included a clinical nurse specialist who was a master of helping people through the grieving process. Following much thinking, the decision was made to have Bill say good-bye to his mother. He would never see her again.

The mother was in the morgue and had to be brought back so he could be with her. The nurse asked the assistant to go to the morgue and pick up the body and bring it back upstairs. He said he couldn't. "We take them to the morgue; we never bring them back!" She explained the situation and he walked away saying, "Boy, things are always changing around here. I'll go, but it is your neck." Yes, it was her neck. She brought the mother into the room and he said good-bye. Did it matter? Will it matter for the rest of his life? The note he wrote to the nurse after leaving the hospital speaks to that. He said, "Thanks for being with me

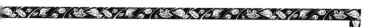

when I said good-bye to my mom."

There was something this emergency room nurse said that still rings in my ear. "I am starting to understand the difference between nursing and medicine, medical care, absence of disease, and health care: body, mind, and spirit in balance. Do you know, if I had never intervened with his grief, nothing would have been said to me. No one would have asked about his grief. No one would have thought less of me. They know I am a good nurse. However, if I had failed to give a medicine that was ordered, there would have been an incident report written. I wonder about the significance of that?" It is something for all of us to think about.

CONSTRUCTING NEW ROADS - THE INTERCHANGE

"The greatest good you can do for another is not just to share your riches, but to reveal to him his own."
- Benjamin Disraeli

Core Belief: **Health care is coordinated and delivered in partnership with the person receiving care.**

This core belief speaks to the critical role nurses play in the health care of this society. Nurses are the coordinators of care. It makes sense, they are the ones providing hands on care and know the person's needs. Some call them case managers, primary nurses, facilitators, or coordinators. It doesn't matter what they are called.

The accountability for the coordination of care sits with the registered nurse. The society's hope for health care and partnership rests in the hands of the person coordinating care. This core belief says that the nurse will always coordinate care in partnership with the person and also within a health care paradigm. This assures the person that they have control over their own health, their own destiny.

Coordinating "absence of disease" is very different than coordinating health: "body, mind, and spirit in balance." Under the medical and institutional care paradigm activities are provided according to the doctor's orders, physical needs, and common physiological progression and treatment patterns. The accountability for coordinating in a medical model evolves around checking to see if things are done on day one, day two, or day three as expected.

Coordination within the medical

framework is based on the typical physical progression and standard treatments for the person's medical condition. It only addresses one basic component of quality, that is, the competency of a synchronized team. However, this core belief calls for coordination within the health care paradigm and in partnership with the person receiving care. It is the phase of quality care that Donabeidan (1980, 1982) refers to as individualized and mutually determined.

Coordination and partnership parallel with the principles of quality. To give quality care Donabedian (1980, 1982) notes the service should be individualized and mutually determined. What does that mean? The word individualized is a common word used by nurses. It is an interesting word and its Latin root means "indivisible." The only way to individualize care is to see the person in his/her wholeness: body, mind, and spirit. We do not heal a person; that is the person's work.

Healing must start within the

person, not just within their arm, leg, chest, or abdomen, but within their wholeness. We can have all the knowledge humanly possible about the body, but that is not enough. We can do everything we want to the body, but in the end, it is only the person's ability to create harmony of body, mind, and spirit that will determine his/her healing. Our role is to support the person on his/her healing journey. The person must take an active, not a passive role. Although healing is the work of the one who is ill, nursing can support the healing process by providing care that is specific to that individual.

The provider must be in synchrony with the person. The nurse needs to be a master of mutuality, which precedes individualization. Mutuality is an ongoing process wherein the nurse seeks to find out from the person what is important for their present and future health status, not just the medical status. It is the first step in developing the mission, the reason for the partnership to exist. Mutuality drives the coordination of health care for the whole team and focuses the necessary care and teaching on the individual's unique needs.

Wisdom From The Field

The following clinical scenarios will show the difference between coordination of care within old and new patterns of thinking. The importance of the role of partnership with the people we serve and the difference between medical and health coordination of care is evident.

Clinical Scenario One: This is about Matt's story as discussed in the previous core belief. The nurse caring for Matt recognized his spiritual distress. She then took action to treat it. Her plan was to bring together the health care team and Matt's significant others to talk about his health situation. She, with the help of a peer, called the interdisciplinary team, significant others, and priest to come to a conference. She also called the physician. She had an excellent professional relationship with this physician. However, she had never called him with a situation like this.

The phone conversation went like this. "I'm calling about Matt to see if we can change the scheduled cervical fusion surgery and halo placement." He wondered why. She told him Matt was in crisis with spiritual distress. There was a pause and he said to her, "Are his vital signs OK?" She noted they were and then he said to her, "What in the hell is spiritual distress?" He later said, in his mind he was thinking, spiritual distress sounds like something to do with God and he didn't want to buck God, but it didn't make a lot of sense to him. The nurse explained that she didn't think it would be good for Matt to go to surgery not wanting to live, having no purpose. She was putting together a conference so as to gain greater insight and consistency on his care at this time. She noted that in the long run it would not delay his progression, but enhance it.

His response was, "I can't." She

wondered why not and he said, "Because, I am going on vacation." She asked if there was someone else who could do it. He asked his partner to do the surgery. Did it matter?

Before this event, Matt had a plan of care that was based on his story given by his significant others on admission. The team had learned that Matt was a quiet person, very academic, disciplined, and although he liked to solve his own problems, he was not an isolationist. His mother noted, "If you ask him about an issue and he snaps at you, you will know two things. One, he snapped because he is concerned about the issue; and two, he is not ready to talk with you about it."

At the scene of his accident, before Matt was intubated, he asked the flight nurse not to take off the cross around his neck. That did not surprise the family who said he found great comfort in his religion, but he was very private about it. Matt's plan of care supported his typical coping patterns. The family would pray daily around his bed, and when the priest came, they would gather again and pray.

During the conference, the nurse shared with the family and inter-disciplinary team Matt's response. He was angry, threw his cross across the room and wondered where God was when he needed him. Matt stated that running was his life and he had no purpose to live. His mother found this situation hopeless. The nurse said it was not hopeless, but a response that is often seen, and in time will resolve. She explained that was why they were meeting, to explore ways to support Matt during this difficult time.

His father referred back to a comment that he shared with the staff on admission about Matt not sharing what was bothering him, unless he was ready. He said he was always impressed with his wife because she seemed to know what was on Matt's mind before he would talk about it.

Matt's mom responded by saying, "That is no big deal. I'll never forget the day we brought his new puppy home.

He talked differently with the dog than anyone else." She said if she was in the basement and she heard Matt talking with the dog, she would come and listen. "He always works things through by talking with his dog before talking with anyone else. That is why I know what is on his mind."

This was new information, an unknown, but important part of his story that reflected one of his critical coping patterns. The nurse made arrangements for the dog to be brought to the hospital. Did it matter? Just a note about bringing the dog into ICU. The dog can be brought into the hospital. Do you know what needs to be done to make that happen?

The dog cried and cried when he came into Matt's room. When things finally calmed down, Matt said to the dog; "Well, we make a great team, you have hip dysplasia and I will never run again." Matt cried. So did everyone in the room. This was the first time Matt cried. Do you think it was hard being with Matt at that moment? Do you see

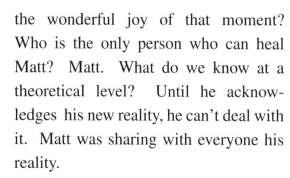

the wonderful joy of that moment?
Who is the only person who can heal
Matt? Matt. What do we know at a
theoretical level? Until he acknow-
ledges his new reality, he can't deal with
it. Matt was sharing with everyone his
reality.

We cannot fix things for Matt.
This core belief speaks clearly about the
shift from fixing, to being present and
intervening to support his healing
journey. The nurse caring for Matt
understood the importance of partnership. Caring is the willingness to stop
fixing and go into partnership with the
person.

Instead of unilaterally making
decisions, she went back to Matt. She
reminded him of the plan of care and
asked if today would be OK for the
family to pray around his bed. He said,
"Yes, they can pray, but I'm not." The
nurse asked, "What about your priest,
would you like him to visit today?" He
said, "Yes, and when he comes, I need to
be alone with him." The nurse noted
his words felt like being hit with a cold

glass of water in the face. He had never been alone with his priest. Yet they knew from his story that he was private, especially about his faith. It was just something that was known about him, but not incorporated into his daily care.

He then asked to talk with his brother, who was outside of the country and he said, "When you get hold of him, I need to be alone with him." Matt's life long patterns of coping were evident.

During the professional exchange report at the conclusion of the shift, the nurse mentioned to the next colleague that Matt was making great inroads, moving along well on his healing journey. This was evident in Matt's decision making. The important point to note here is why? *Because Matt was given a choice.*

The nurse was establishing partnership with Matt. Mutuality was at the center of the relationship. That is a practice pattern of the new paradigms, not of the old. In this situation, there was no policy, procedure, medication or medical treatment that could have replaced the nurse's intervention to optimize Matt's health. It was driven from a different understanding, a different knowledge base. It is very different from the following scenario.

Clinical Scenario Two: George was a 50 year old man in love with life. When he was diagnosed with cancer, his world instantly changed. He was not afraid of dying. He just wanted to live. He had two sons and a loving wife. He had shared with a nurse friend that he was concerned about his youngest son, Jeff, who would not talk about his dad's life threatening situation. George's hope was for his sons to experience joy in their lives. He was wise and knew that joy would hinge on the ability of his sons to experience a healthy grieving process. George ended up getting an infection and dying sooner than anticipated.

At the funeral home, the nurse friend was standing by a picture of George when his son Jeff approached. He had left the receiving line to talk with her. At one point in the conversation the nurse asked him if he had a chance to say good-bye to his father. He said yes, he was sorry it took so long and that his dad had to suffer so much. Then he said, "I was so angry." The nurse immediately made an assumption that his anger was related to his father's death, a common stage of grief. That was not accurate. He then said, "I was so angry with the nurse." The nurse was troubled and asked what happened.

Jeff started by making excuses for the nurse, not saying what happened. It went something like this. "Maybe she was right. I have been thinking about when it happened. It happened right after they told us dad probably would die in the next few hours. Mom didn't think so because she thought he would wait until his friend got there and he was coming from a long ways."

George had made it known that he wanted his death to be like his father's. George's father died while his family was gathered around his bed, holding hands, praying, and singing. He talked about how that was so good for

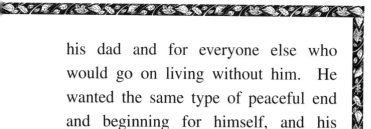

his dad and for everyone else who would go on living without him. He wanted the same type of peaceful end and beginning for himself, and his family and friends.

Jeff then said, "I think it happened just after everyone had finally arrived. Yes, everyone was there. Maybe she was right. There were probably 25 of us gathered around dad's bed. It was pretty crowded. That is when she came in and said, "There are too many people in here. Only the immediate family and a couple others can be here!"" He said, "I was so angry."

What about you nurse? What are you feeling at this moment? What do you think about this situation? You may be thinking, I never would have done that. It doesn't matter what you would do, it matters what any of us would do.

The nurse friend was touched intensely by the wisdom of this young man. Jeff said, "The reason I was so angry was because we didn't have a choice, and the way in which it was done." There was no mutuality and therefore, could be no individualization nor partnership. This is a violation of the core beliefs of professional nursing. However, this practice is a norm in hospitals across this country, a practice rooted in the old paradigms.

Here are some thoughts to ponder. What does it mean to practice partnership in a health care paradigm? What does it mean to coordinate care within this paradigm? What is the nurse's role?

Some of the most important nursing care given happens during what Leland Kaiser (1994) refers to as the "deathing" process for one person and the continuation of life for the person's significant others. What does it mean in a practical sense that the presence of the nurse should bring hope and light to any situation? Is partnership the first step of hope, and the coordination of health care the light?

CONSTRUCTING NEW ROADS -
THE BYPASS

"It is not so much that we're afraid of change, or so in love with the old ways, but it's that place in between we fear.....it's like being in between trapezes. It's Linus when his blanket is in the dryer. There is nothing to hold on to."

- Marilyn Ferguson

Core Belief: **New ways of thinking are essential to continually improve health care throughout the life span.**

$\mathcal{F}$or the body to live, it must change everyday. If it doesn't, it will die. What about the mind and spirit? It was only the limitations of our minds, notes Fox (1958), that prevented the development of electricity, television, air, space travel, and other advances much sooner in our history. They were possible, but the limits were in the minds and thinking of the people at that time. What else is there that we cannot see because of the limits of our minds, our thinking? The challenge is to free our minds, shed our paradigms, and constantly be vigilant to new thinking. We only stay in a paradigm so we can actualize the potential of that paradigm while readying ourselves for newer thinking. It is traveling without baggage.

Old patterns naturally lead to new patterns unless we cling, defend, and protect the old patterns. See Figure 7, which visually shows that evolution. We need to become comfortable with transition. Life is nothing more than a journey from one paradigm to the next. If we cannot let go of the old, there is no journey; it is a continuous ride on the carousel. If we can't let go, then we cannot continuously learn. If we become comfortable with black and white, then gray, or continuous learning,

FIGURE 7

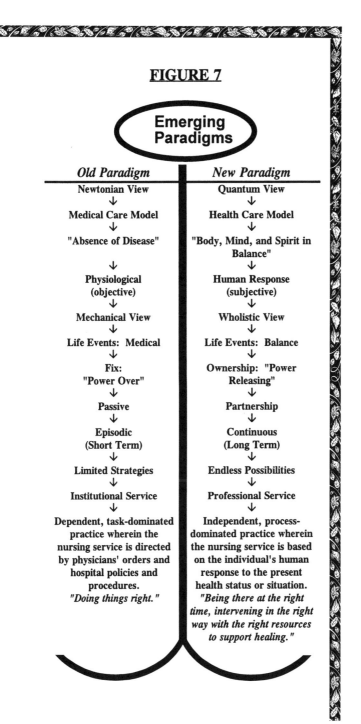

Emerging Paradigms

Old Paradigm	*New Paradigm*
Newtonian View	Quantum View
↓	↓
Medical Care Model	Health Care Model
↓	↓
"Absence of Disease"	"Body, Mind, and Spirit in Balance"
↓	↓
Physiological (objective)	Human Response (subjective)
↓	↓
Mechanical View	Wholistic View
↓	↓
Life Events: Medical	Life Events: Balance
↓	↓
Fix: "Power Over"	Ownership: "Power Releasing"
↓	↓
Passive	Partnership
↓	↓
Episodic (Short Term)	Continuous (Long Term)
↓	↓
Limited Strategies	Endless Possibilities
↓	↓
Institutional Service	Professional Service
↓	↓
Dependent, task-dominated practice wherein the nursing service is directed by physicians' orders and hospital policies and procedures. *"Doing things right."*	Independent, process-dominated practice wherein the nursing service is based on the individual's human response to the present health status or situation. *"Being there at the right time, intervening in the right way with the right resources to support healing."*

becomes stressful, instead of joyful.

Staying in an old paradigm can prevent learning and new thinking. Without new thinking there is no chance for improvement of health care. How sad, how hopeless. For some it may be hopeless or sad because of the system's present reality, but for others it is sad or hopeless because of the loss of potential for what the system could become. If we choose not to change our minds, what has been is all there will be.

What is there about our minds that causes us to hesitate with change? Fox (1958) states, "The history of scientific discovery shows that almost every new step was opposed by the very people who should welcome it." Ferguson (1980) thought it was fear. She describes fear as that space, or time, between trapezes when there is nothing to hang on to before catching the other trapeze. Is this fear of the unknown or truth? The mind, one's thinking, can prevent one from ever letting go. The body is at the command of the mind. It cannot let go or hang on.

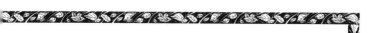

The expression, the potential of the spirit can also be limited by the mind. Our thinking can prevent the spirit from having the opportunity to help us fly from one trapeze to the other. It was the mind and spirit that gave Matt wings when his legs and feet no longer worked. The spirit is the potential of every human being. It is the invisible, intangible, immaterial domain of every human that is connected to every other human and to the Ultimate Spirit. The mind and the spirit in partnership provide unlimited support for transitions. When we hold on to old thinking and do not continuously learn, our spirit, our potential, is trapped within.

Transition from old to new patterns of thinking has been difficult for this present culture. New thinking is nothing more than new learning. Somewhere along the line our present society started to see the learning process as one with a beginning and an end. No more trapezes to grab on to.

That is evident in the education

system. We even ask people, "At what point did you end your education: high school, college, masters, Ph.D., or post doctoral? Where did you end your learning?"

In practice we talk about ending orientation, getting checked off on treatments, achieving credentialing, going back for another degree, getting the continued education credits for the year. Learning is another task to be done. It is seen as a task that takes place in a certain space, such as schools, skills labs, classes or within a period of time. The greatest gift a teacher could give another is help on how to become a master in transition from old to new patterns of thinking.

Learning and new thinking have no end, only beginnings. New thinking in the mind unlocks the door to endless possibilities because it frees up the spirit. Health care and nursing are only limited in our minds.

The health care setting is no exception to the segmented concept of learning and practice. It is easy to see

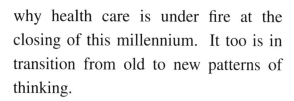

why health care is under fire at the closing of this millennium. It too is in transition from old to new patterns of thinking.

Work was begun twelve years ago in a community based midwestern hospital to change the nursing department from a fragmented, unit focused, specialty focused mentality to a systems thinking department. The need for new thinking is evident in the following scenario.

Wisdom From The Field

Clinical Scenario: An elderly gentleman named Frank had been diagnosed with Alzheimer's. His thinking was no longer clear enough for him to be alone and safe, so he was placed in a foster care facility. The family had shared his story with the people in the facility and they knew him well.

Frank needed to come to the emergency room because he had fallen and lost consciousness for a short time. While in the emergency room, he was interviewed by the admitting nurse, a medical student, the medical resident, the neuroresident, and the attending physician. He was transferred to the neuro unit and was interviewed by the unit nurse. He was not capable of answering most of the questions, but felt the responsibility to respond in his limited capacity.

During the interview on the neuro unit, he looked at his family member and said, "Don't they talk with each other?" The family was amazed, because it wasn't often he used complete sentences and even then the appropriateness of most of his responses were often questionable. However, this confused person had enough sense to question the way things were being done. How many times have you asked a person a question about their history or story, a question that was asked by another health care provider somewhere else along the road? Why do we continue these patterns?

Agreeing that we ought to change the system will not make it happen.

This core belief gives clear direction. Practice, or the way we deliver our service, will not change until we change our thinking. It is not just the individual provider who must change. It is more than that. It involves a system or structure change as well. It can be achieved if the providers become systems thinkers. Senge (1990) defines systems thinking as, "Discipline of understanding the dynamic rather than the detail complexity of systems, seeing the whole, interrelationships, and patterns of change." It requires new ways of thinking.

Frank's health is not about this one event. This event is only part of his health picture. The health care paradigm calls for the providers to know his story, it does not call for the person to tell his story over and over again, and again, and again. The pattern will be changed only when the providers agree to change their day to day rituals and patterns

In Frank's case, it calls for the providers in the nursing facility to connect with the providers in the emergency department, and for them to connect with the neuro unit, etc. Unless the providers change to a systems thinking approach for care and reach out to each other across settings and within settings, it will not happen. This requires new thinking, new learning.

Is it work to change thinking? Recall one bad habit you have. Have you tried to change this bad habit? Were you successful with the change and thought you finally licked it, when all of a sudden you are right back doing it again? Do you know at a personal level how hard it is to change a habit? That is how hard it is to change thinking that is linked to the daily rituals and patterns of practice that are older than all of us.

The following key learning has emerged throughout the twelve years of work to support living the core beliefs. The practice culture, as well as the design of the system and structures will impact the individual's work to change from old to new thinking. The learnings from this work are immense and will be the focus of another book in this series.

CONSTRUCTING NEW ROADS - AN AIRFIELD.

"You are the problem, the solution, the resource."
                                    - Leland Kaiser

Core belief: **Empowerment begins with each person and is enhanced by relationships and systems design.**

*E*mpowerment is most commonly defined as "one with authority or power." Some think that in an empowered culture, everyone has the authority or power to act as one individually desires. That is not empowerment, that is anarchy. *Empowerment is a state of being in which the person, the nurse, has the* *power, the authority to act in his/her role to achieve the mission and live the core beliefs.* It is something that happens inside the person. It cannot be measured at the material level since it is about the mind, and spirit, or will. It has to do with the immaterial strength of the individual, as nurse.

This belief brings a powerful message that we believe each person, whether provider or recipient of care, is accountable for, and has ownership of his/her own life, health, healing, and mission. The peace, joy, adventure, love, fun and balance in life depends on our thinking. How we choose to think determines our destiny.

Although empowerment starts within the individual, it is enhanced by relationships with others, the systems, and cultures. It is about the bottom "R," relationships, a leverage point for a successful journey. Relationships, as health care, go beyond the physical to the intangible mind and spirit connections.

The goal in most health care

settings is to improve the quality of health care services. The quality of care cannot be improved until the relationships between health care providers and the people they are privileged to serve, as well as the practice systems, are improved. There is a problem when providers allow someone to interfere with their ability to carry out the mission and core beliefs. As Leland Kaiser (1994) notes the problem begins within the individual. The solution and resource to end that problem also rests within the individual.

Relationships and systems that enhance the empowerment of the nurse, the recipients of care, and every health care provider, are very different than the typical bureaucratic and hierarchical systems found in many practice settings. The work and learning over the last twelve years, to live this core belief, are so important that they will be the focus of the next book in this series. The wisdom from the field will flow from the many rural, community, and university settings that have come together to create empowered cultures where individual ownership and accountability to mission, team integration, innovation, and partnership are transforming individuals and health care settings.

A REASON TO CONTINUE

"There are truths which belong to the future, truths which belong to the past, and truths which belong to no time."
                                    - Carl Gustav Jung

I wonder if the work of clarifying our core beliefs with dialogue and discussion is only the search for the truths which belong to no time? If core beliefs are the foundation for the journey, it seems we would want them to be of a timeless nature. At least we hope we are pushing on the truths of tomorrow that will lead on to the truths that belong to no time, but all time. Whatever, clarifying core beliefs is important work. The work is to align our beliefs that guide our work with the highest level of truth. Truth that transcends not only individual wisdom but collective wisdom.

A journey without core beliefs might be compared to taking an airplane that does not have flight instrumentation. When the snow, rain, or fog hits, there is no visualization and numerous planes are traveling the same skies and coming in to the same airports. The radio waves safely direct the pilot across the skies and assist with a safe landing. It decreases the anxieties during major weather changes. It also takes away the unnecessary worry of what to do "if" bad weather happens. It does not change the weather. Core beliefs are like flight instrumentation. They assist us as we travel through the fog, the storms of these times. So whether it be snow, sleet, mergers, managed care, or national health insurance, we will be able to continue our travels with an assurance far beyond the changing winds.

What is the importance of core beliefs? They help us know our similarities as nurses. The understanding of similarities frees us to see and respect our diversity while developing our profession and the health of this society. Emile Durkhelm noted that, "When mores are sufficient, laws are unnecessary. When mores are insufficient, laws are unenforceable." So it is with core beliefs. When core beliefs are sufficient, we are released from the jaws of rituals, patterns and routines of institutional nursing and there is hope for consistency on things that matter most.

Consistency of core beliefs is essential. It is strengthened by diversity of thinking. Diversity of thinking and opinion stimulates the dialogue that leads to a deeper understanding of the core beliefs, the essence of health, the essence of nursing. Clarity of the core beliefs keeps us in touch with things that matter most and energizes us during chaos.

Depree (1992) stated, "Change without continuity is chaos. Continuity without change is sloth and very risky." Core beliefs give us continuity with flexible boundaries, so we can move out of chaos into a higher order. The real challenge we face is not saying what we believe; it is in living what we believe. Inconsistency in the living of the core beliefs surrounds us. The majority of nurses in the United States practice in the hospital where institutional nursing became a form of continuity. That is risky.

In the beginning I promised a glimpse into the future. So here it is. If you go back and look at the comments you made in the columns, you will see the future. It will be everything you thought it would be! I hope you will take the time to share that with me. If so, please send it to the CPM Resource Center. See the Appendix, pages 167 - 169, for information.

Our journey from old to new ways of thinking, to new ways of practice, is just beginning. Winston Churchill's words ring with truth about where we are at this moment, "This is not the end, this is not the beginning of the end, but perhaps it is the end of the beginning." We have ended the

Bibliography

American Nurses Association (1980). <u>Nursing: A social policy statement</u>. Kansas City: The American Nurses Association.

American Nurses Association (1995). <u>Nursing: A social policy statement</u>. Washington, DC: The American Nurses Association.

Barker, J. (1990). <u>The business of paradigms: Discovering the future</u>. (Video Cassette) Burnsville, MN: Charthouse International Learning Corporation.

Bohm, D. (1983). <u>Wholeness and the implicate order</u>. London: Ark Paperbacks.

Covey, S. (1990). <u>Principle-centered leadership</u>. New York: Simon & Schuster.

DePree, M. (1992). <u>Leadership jazz</u>. New York: Doubleday.

Donabedian, A. (1982). <u>The criteria and standards of quality</u>. Ann Arbor: Health Administration Press.

Donabedian, A. (1980). <u>The definition of quality and approaches to its assessment</u>. Ann Arbor: Health Administration Press.

Einstein, A. (1993). <u>Einstein in humanism</u>. New York: Acitated Press Book.

Ferguson, M. (1980). <u>The aquarian conspiracy</u>. Los Angeles: J.P. Tarchert, Inc.

Fox, E. (1958). <u>Around the year with Emmet Fox</u>. San Francisco: Harper Collins Publisher.

Fox, E. (1941). <u>Find and use your inner power</u>. San Francisco: Harper Collins Publisher.

Hart, P. (1990). <u>A nationwide survey of attitudes toward health care and nurses</u>. Washington, D.C.: Peter Hart Research Associates, Inc.

Kaiser, L. (Speaker). (1994). <u>Creating the future of health care</u>. (Cassette recording No. 94-3401). Front Royal, VA: National Cassette Services, Inc.

Maloney, Mary (1992). <u>Professionalization of nursing, current issues and trends</u>. Philadelphia: J.B. Lippincott Co.

Naisbitt, J. & Aburdene, P. (1982). <u>Megatrends</u>. New York: William Marrow.

Nightingale, Florence (1859). <u>Notes on nursing</u>. Philadelphia: J.B. Lippincott.

Nouwen, H. (1974). <u>Out of solitude</u>. Notre Dame, IN: Ave Maria Press.

Peat, F.P. (1993). <u>Lighting the seventh fire</u>. New York: U Birch Lane Press Book.

Roach, S. (1991). Response to: "Being There: Who do you bring to practice?" In Gaut, D. (Ed.), <u>The presence of caring in nursing</u>. New York: National League for Nursing Press.

Senge, P. (1990). <u>The fifth discipline: The art and practice of the learning organization</u>. New York: Doubleday/Currency.

Ulrich, B. (1992). <u>Leadership and management according to Florence Nightingale</u>. Norwalk: Appleton and Lange.

Underwood, P. (1993). <u>The walking people, a native american oral history</u>. San Ansel Mo, CA: A Tribe of Two Press.

Wesorick, B. (1990). <u>Standards of nursing care: A model for clinical practice</u>. Philadelphia: J.B. Lippincott Co.

Wheatley, M. (1993). <u>Leadership and the new science</u>. San Francisco: Berrett-Koehler Publisher.

APPENDIX A

Clinical Practice Model (CPM) Resource Center
Grand Rapids, Michigan

Mission
Enhance partnering relationships and world linkages for generation of collective knowledge and wisdom that continually improves the structure, process and outcomes of professional nursing and community health care services.

Bonnie Wesorick, RN, MSN, *President*
Laurie Shiparski, RN, BSN, MS, *Professional Practice Consultant*
Diane Hanson, RN, MSN, *Practice Guidelines Specialist*
Darlene Josephs, CPS, *Operations Administrator*
Linda Schagel, *Administrative Secretary*

Researchers:
Karen Grigsby, RN, PhD
Donna Westmoreland, RN, PhD
University of Nebraska Medical Center
College of Nursing, Omaha, Nebraska

CPM Resource Center Associate Consortium
Mission: Collectively create professional practice and learning environments that empower each partner to provide their unique healing contribution.

Linda Engdahl, RN, MS
Carmen Hall, RNC, BS, MA
Mary Koloroutis, RN, MS
Abbott Northwestern Hospital
Minneapolis, Minnesota

Michelle Troseth, RN, BSN
Bonnie Wesorick, RN, MSN, Senior Advisor for Professional Practice
Kathy Wyngarden, RN, MSN
Butterworth Hospital
Grand Rapids, Michigan

Cindy Simons, RN, BSN
Ambulatory Butterworth
Grand Rapids, Michigan

Dee Blakey, RN, BSN
Flagstaff Medical Center
Flagstaff, Arizona

Betty Jo Balzar, RN, BSN
Appleton Medical Center
Appleton, Wisconsin

Brenda Srof, RN, MSN
Goshen College
Goshen, Indiana

Dorinda Leonard, RN
Harris Continued Care
Hospital
Fort Worth, Texas

Connie McAllister, RN,
MSN
Liberty Hospital
Liberty, Missouri

Joan Schulz, RN
Harris Continued Care
Hospital - HEB
Bedford, Texas

Crystal Beresford, RN,
BSN, CRRN
Macomb Hospital Center
Warren, Michigan

Rochelle Jee, RN
Harris Methodist
Southwest
Fort Worth, Texas

Linda Barnes, RN, BS
Magic Valley Regional
Medical Center
Twin Falls, Idaho

Marsha Vanderveen, RN,
MSN
Holland Community
Hospital
Holland, Michigan

Shirley Hamann, RN,
MSN
Medcenter One
Bismarck, North Dakota

Beth Adams, RN
Home Health Care
Holland, Michigan

Amy Horst
Medical College of Ohio
Hospital
Toledo, Ohio

Cheryl Doherty, RN
Hotel Dieu Grace Hospital
Crawford Site
Windsor, Ontario Canada

Cathy Schwartz, RN, MS
Memorial Medical Center
Springfield, Illinois

Barbara Scarpelli, RN,
BScN
Hotel Dieu Grace Hospital
Ouellette Site
Windsor, Ontario Canada

M.J. Petersen, RN, MSN
Mercy Hospital
Council Bluffs, Iowa

Linda Dietrich, RN, MSN
Kaiser Sunnyside Hospital
Clackamas, Oregon

Pat Nakoneczny, RN, BSN
Northern Michigan
Hospital
Petoskey, Michigan

Carol Robinson, RN, MS, CNA
Phoenix Children's Hospital
Phoenix, Arizona

Lynn Hollister, RNC, MS
St. Mark's Hospital
Salt Lake City, Utah

Peggy Flores, RN
Providence Memorial Hospital
El Paso, Texas

Sandy Panzer, RN, MSN
Theda Clark Regional Medical Center
Neenah, Wisconsin

Ernie Fuller, RN, BSN
Saint Joseph Health Center
Kansas City, Missouri

Rani Srivastava, RN, MScN
Wellesley Hospital
Toronto, Ontario

Deb Zielenski
St. Jude Medical Center
Fullerton, California

Susan Boohar, RN, BSN
Wesley Medical Center
Wichita, Kansas

Send feedback on core beliefs or any comments or inquiries regarding this journey to:

CPM Resource Center
100 Michigan Street
Grand Rapids, MI 49503
(616) 776-2017
(616) 456-2770 FAX

"THOUGHTS"